SCIENTIFIC AMERICAN EXPLORES BIG IDEAS

Understanding Cancer

The Editors of *Scientific American*

SCIENTIFIC AMERICAN EDUCATIONAL PUBLISHING

New York

Published in 2024 by Scientific American Educational Publishing
in association with **The Rosen Publishing Group**
2544 Clinton Street, Buffalo NY 14224

Contains material from Scientific American®, a division of Springer Nature America, Inc., reprinted by permission, as well as original material from The Rosen Publishing Group®.

First Edition

Scientific American
Lisa Pallatroni: Project Editor

Rosen Publishing
Michael Hessel-Mial: Compiling Editor
Michael Moy: Senior Graphic Designer

Cataloging-in-Publication Data
Names: Scientific American Editors (New York, New York), editor.
Title: Understanding cancer / Scientific American Editors.
Other titles: Understanding cancer (Scientific American Educational Publishing)
Description: First edition. | Buffalo, NY : Scientific American Educational Publishing, 2024. | Series: Scientific American explores big ideas | Includes bibliographical references and index. | Audience: Grades 10-12
Identifiers: LCCN 2023036932 | ISBN 9781725350281 (library binding) | ISBN 9781725350274 (paperback)| ISBN 9781725350298 (ebook)
Subjects: LCSH: Cancer–Juvenile literature.
Classification: LCC RC264 .U53 2024 | DDC 616.99/4–dc23/eng/20230817
LC record available at https://lccn.loc.gov/2023036932

Manufactured in the United States of America
Websites listed were live at the time of publication.

Cover: SciePro/Shutterstock.com

CPSIA Compliance Information: Batch # CWSA24.
For Further Information contact Rosen Publishing at 1-800-237-9932.

CONTENTS

INTRODUCTION

As the second leading cause of death in the world, cancer impacts nearly everyone. Many of us know someone who has lost a relative or friend to the disease, or who has struggled with its painful treatment. Cancer is also unique for its origin in our own bodies, as rebel cells overtake a patient's organs or tissues. With such a common tragedy following different rules from viruses or bacteria, it makes sense that cancer would earn so much scientific attention. Coming into the 21st century, the causes and treatment of cancer were well established. Cancer emerges due to mutations in cellular DNA. It is typically treated with surgical tissue removal, plus chemotherapy and radiation to destroy further cancerous cells.

Fortunately, recent research has introduced radical new understandings of cancer, which this volume will explore in five sections. The first section covers basic cancer research: its causes, new research into tumors, and new patterns of its appearance in human populations. The second section explores testing, from research into non-invasive early detection of cancer, to the gaps in testing that lead people to get late-stage diagnoses. The third section details cancer prevention; along with the surprising role of sleep hygiene in cancer risk, we learn about novel vaccine developments that might prevent the disease from taking hold. The fourth section concerns cancer treatment, which has shown some of the most exciting advances. Immunotherapy and novel approaches to chemotherapy are among the most promising developments. Lastly, the fifth section concerns the social and ethical dimensions of cancer. Social inequities lead to cancer inequities too, and these articles raise important questions about the accessibility of testing and care.

Cancer is often personal. It might seem that the often impersonal work of scientific research might not honor the anxiety and grief that cancer causes. But as you read, you'll find that the personal stories of patients, loved ones, and passionate researchers reveal the human stories behind this often deadly phenomenon.

Section 1: Novel Cancer Research

Cancerous Coconspirators: Tumor Cells That Travel Together Spread Cancer

By Viviane Callier

Metastasis is behind the vast majority of cancer deaths: when cancer cells break away from a tumor and lodge in new places, the disease becomes harder to treat. A new study shows that, contrary to expectations, most metastatic tumors are seeded not by single cells from the primary tumor but by clusters of diverse cancer cells that leave in a group and travel through the bloodstream together. The cells in these circulating clusters communicate with one another and produce specific proteins that could be used as drug targets or biomarkers for risk of metastasis.

To determine how metastases form, cancer cell biologist Andrew Ewald and his team at Johns Hopkins University created tumors in mice by injecting a mixture of multicolored cancer cells into the rodents' mammary glands. If tumors originated elsewhere from single cells, then they would show up under the microscope as one uniform color. If instead tumors were seeded by clusters of cells, then they would grow into rainbow-colored balls. The team found that about 95 percent of the cancers that formed were in fact multicolored and therefore derived from multiple cells.

In a second experiment, the researchers examined hundreds of cancerous cells grown together in a petri dish but placed so that they were not touching. Almost all of them died. In contrast, cells in another dish that were aggregated into clusters subsequently formed more colonies–even though there were fewer "seeds" to begin with. "Controlling for cell number, there is more than a 100-fold increase in efficiency of metastasis formation in the aggregated cells," Ewald says. The findings were published in February in the *Proceedings of the National Academy of Sciences USA*.

It is not yet entirely clear why the aggregated cells survive and metastasize more effectively, but it is likely that cooperation among tumor cells within clusters—for example, exchanging signaling molecules—protects against cell death in the bloodstream or at distant sites, explains Joan Brugge, a cancer cell biologist at Harvard Medical School who was not involved in the study.

As for potential benefits to patients, Ewald's team also found that the traveling clusters share molecular features and nearly all make the protein keratin 14. "We could potentially use this [insight] to develop targeted ways to attack all the metastatic cells," Ewald says. The idea would be to wipe out those cells wherever they are in the body, whether or not they are proliferating—a different approach from most standard therapies, which focus on attacking rapidly proliferating cells but not the circulating, invasive ones that initiate secondary cancers.

About the Author

Viviane Callier is a freelance science writer based in North Bethesda, Md.

Close-Up Views of Tumors Reveal a New Cancer Biology

By Philip Ball

When Brad Bernstein first looked at cancer tumors cell by cell in 2014, what he found dismayed him: he realized that in any single tumor, there is not one type of cancer cell at work but many. "I was a little depressed when I saw it," says Bernstein, a pathologist at the Broad Institute of the Massachusetts Institute of Technology and Harvard University. "Some of the toughest tumors out there are really heterogeneous mixtures [of cells]."

But for many clinicians and surgeons working to treat cancer, this observation about the nature of tumor cells was a glass more half-full than half-empty. They already knew that treating some tumors is an incredibly difficult problem, Bernstein says, "and now you've shed light on *why* it's an incredibly difficult problem."

In order to zoom in and look at a tumor one cell at a time, Bernstein and his colleagues use a technique called single-cell RNA sequencing (scRNA seq). It shows, in principle, what each individual cell in a sample is doing and which genes within that cell are active. This technology is revealing a whole new dimension to cancerous tumors–that they are mosaics of different cell types, more like loosely structured organs than an undisciplined mass of replicating cells, as was previously thought. And these tumor cells can change their developmental path in a fluid manner, presenting unique challenges–and opportunities–for treatment.

Six years after Bernstein and his team got that initial up-close view, scRNA seq has become recognized as one of the most powerful new approaches in cell biology. Two types of RNA are the intermediary molecules that help translate genes into proteins, so their presence in a cell indicates that a corresponding gene is active. It is now possible to separate and identify the sequence of nearly every RNA in a given cell so rapidly that thousands of cells can be analyzed at once in a tissue sample.

The technique can, for example, show researchers how the body's development unfolds step by step in minute detail as cells differentiate from an initial stem cell state (in which they are capable of becoming any tissue type) and acquire their final "fate" in a particular tissue. When used to analyze tumors, scRNA seq has revealed that cancer is not simply a breakdown of the developmental process, a glitch that produces rogue, uncontrolled cell proliferation.

Instead, Bernstein says, "we're learning that a brain tumor is sort of like a deranged recapitulation of normal development." Single-cell RNA sequencing "opens your eyes to what is actually in the tumor," he adds, "and the answer is: a lot more than tumor cells." Tumors are not masses of identical cancer cells but a closely bound mixture of many cell types–including plenty of nonmalignant so-called healthy cells. Yet these nonmalignant cells, Bernstein says, "are not innocent bystanders." They seem to help support the tumor somehow.

Though this situation makes the challenge of treating cancers seem more daunting, it could also make treatments ultimately much more effective. If researchers know which of the various types of malignant cells are present, they can tailor a specific cocktail of drugs to attack them. Such detailed information at the single-cell level "is clearly revolutionizing our understanding of cancer," says Mario Suvà of Massachusetts General Hospital. Whereas previous work focused on certain functional properties of single cancer cells or genomics of the whole tumor, Suvà says, researchers are now seeing everything at the cellular level.

For instance, previous studies had seemed to suggest that one of four distinct types of cancer cells might be present in any given brain tumor, creating four different classes of tumor–each needing a different kind of treatment. Bernstein's single-cell analyses of a particularly malignant type of brain tumor called a glioblastoma, however, revealed that *all four* cell types were typically present in every tumor he and his colleagues looked at. But they occurred in different proportions, so only the dominant type tended to be seen in bulk studies. "It was astounding to us," Bernstein says. Rather than four distinct classes of tumor, single-cell analysis showed that there is a continuum of tumor type, each comprised of a mixture of those four malignant cell varieties (typically along with various healthy cells, too).

"We probably need a diagnostic test that could take a tumor and see which of the major cell groups are present," Bernstein says. Researchers would then hit them with so-called combination therapies, which apply several different drug agents at once. Such mixtures are difficult to develop and test, he admits, but in the long run, they could be more effective at mopping up all the dangerous cells.

The different cell types in a tumor arise by differentiation from a kind of cancer "stem cell"—just as normal cells differentiate in ordinary tissues in a developing embryo. "Tumors mostly follow a similar hierarchy of starting in a stemlike state," says Mariella Filbin, a pediatric neuro-oncologist at the Dana-Farber Cancer Institute and Boston Children's Hospital, who has collaborated with Suvà's team. But cancer cells do not quite make it to the usual fates of other cells, Filbin explains. "Some get stuck and just proliferate."

Cancer cell differentiation also seems to be more fluid than that of healthy cells. "It's not like a normal hierarchy, where you differentiate, and then you're committed [to a fate]," Bernstein says. Cancer cells might differentiate a little bit and then revert, he adds. Such reversibility and plasticity create real challenges for therapies that target one cell type: the interchangeability of these states gives cancer cells a survival strategy. "The tumors can become something else and escape our drug therapies," Filbin says. "It's very easy for them."

Another problem is that some tumors might be mostly nonmalignant. In a study of squamous epidermal cancer of the head and neck three years ago, Bernstein and his colleagues learned that one group of patients' tumors had a high number of seemingly ordinary fibroblasts—connective-tissue cells—which were derived from so-called epithelial cells. "Some tumors might just have 5 to 10 percent tumor cells, and the rest are nonmalignant cells sitting in the tumor ecosystem," he says. But such tumors seem to be able to use these cells for malicious ends. In some cases, the healthy epithelial cells turn into earlier-stage mesenchymal cells, break free from the tumor and become mobile in the body. That is, these tumors reinitiate an earlier developmental process to bring about invasive metastasis, dispersing the cancer and making it very hard to treat. "None of this stuff comes out of bulk analysis," Bernstein notes.

The disturbing ability of cancer cells to hijack healthy cells is illustrated in a recent report by Moran Amit of the University of Texas MD Anderson Cancer Center and his colleagues. By looking at the RNA profiles of cells in squamous tumor cells in the head and neck, they found those cancerous cells can reprogram ordinary neurons so that they promote tumor growth.

The new picture of cancer provided by scRNA seq might open possibilities for entirely new treatments. Suvà has used the technique to study tumors' immune system–specifically, the T cells they contain, which are the main agents of our normal immune response. Boosting the immune system has already been found to give it the capacity to attack cancer cells. But doing so has only been effective for certain types of cancer–namely leukemias. Suvà hopes that studying the immune status of tumors might point to new options for such cancer immunotherapies. Looking cell by cell, he says, is "a powerful tool for the discovery of new biology."

The insights this technique has already provided might suggest an even more dramatic cure. The unusual plasticity of cancer cells–which can transition back and forth between different states more readily than normal cells–means that instead of simply trying to kill them, it might be possible to "cure" them by guiding them gently back to a nonmalignant state. This process is called differentiation therapy, and Filbin is hunting for small-molecule drugs that can do it. She and her colleagues are exploring the approach for neuroblastoma, an aggressive form a cancer that afflicts children's nervous system. (The new technique would be used after treatment with conventional chemotherapy and radiotherapy.) And a team in Germany and Italy tried treating a particularly challenging form of leukemia called APML (acute promyelocytic leukaemia) without chemotherapy at all. Instead the researchers only employed two differentiation agents: all-trans retinoic acid and arsenic trioxide. They found a nearly 98 percent survival rate for patients after 50 months. "This is differentiation therapy at its best," Filbin says. She and her colleagues have also found that differentiation can put cancer cells in a senescent state that eventually leads to cell death.

"Right now I'm treating brain tumors where we have nothing: they are resistant to chemo- and radiotherapies," Filbin says. "So we can't seem to kill those cells. But maybe we can differentiate them." If so, she adds, "I'd be the happiest woman on the planet."

About the Author

Philip Ball is a science writer based in London. His book How Life Works *(University of Chicago Press) was published in 2023.*

How Evolution Helps Us Understand Cancer and Control It

By Athena Aktipis

A humpback whale is among the largest animals on this planet, now or ever. It is also a gigantic society made of quadrillions of cooperating cells. Different cell types orchestrate eating, breathing, swimming, reproduction, reacting to other animals, and all the functions that are necessary for a whale to survive and thrive. If you look inside an elephant, a person or even a saguaro cactus, you will see a similarly well-functioning cellular civilization.

Multicellular creatures evolved in the first place because cells that cooperate had advantages over loners such as a single-celled bacterium. Sharing resources allowed life-forms to become larger—a benefit that helps them resist predators—because nutrients and chemical signals that cells need could be transported around the body. Dividing labor let cells specialize and build useful parts such as a stomach or legs. And teamwork gave them the ability to maintain a healthy extracellular environment so they could live longer than they otherwise would.

But cooperation is a fragile proposition. Within multicellular life, cheaters can prosper. By hogging resources, they replicate more quickly than cooperators and take over, unless there are mechanisms to enforce cooperation. Cheating cells can take advantage of the cooperative cellular society they are living in, overproliferating, monopolizing nutrients and otherwise disrupting the harmony that makes multicellular organisms viable in the first place. This cellular cheating is what we know as cancer.

Cancer cells break the rules of normal cells. They divide when they should not, do not die when they should, rob other cells of essential supplies, shirk their cellular jobs and pollute the extracellular space. While cooperating cells curb excess growth and proliferation, cancer cells often evade growth-suppressing signals. Cooperating cells have limited lives, but cancer cells resist cell death and hide from an immune system that would typically destroy them. Normal cells distribute nutrients and chemical signals essential to survival, but cancer cells grow extra blood vessels to grab more resources for themselves. These contrasts show us that cheating is not merely a metaphor for cancer. It is a description of cancer's cellular reality.

This lens of evolution and cooperation is providing scientists with new insights into the way cancer happens—and why it does not. Giant animals such as the whale and elephant, for instance, rarely get cancer despite having multitudes of cells that can go wrong. Why? A number of researchers, including our team at Arizona State University's Arizona Cancer Evolution Center, have examined the genomes of these giants and found they have many copies of genes that destroy cells that mutate and produce aberrant proteins, a signal of cancer. The animals also have extra copies of genes that trigger DNA repair. These genes are, essentially, the cooperation police. One of them, called *TP53*, has been identified as a cancer suppressor in people—but unlike the giant animals, we have only two copies, and unsurprisingly we are more prone to malignancies. Researchers are now trying to translate the actions of such genes into therapies and looking for similar genes all across the tree of life. Oncologists have even started to use evolutionary principles to design chemotherapy that protects less aggressive, less selfish cells within a nascent tumor, reducing the cancer's danger.

The Cooperation Game

I was first drawn to this evolutionary interplay between cooperation and cheating when I was getting my undergraduate and graduate degrees in psychology. I wrote computer programs that tested the effects of different strategies on hypothetical populations, rather like nodes in a network. Generally in such models, without countervailing forces such as genetic relatedness or social norms of reciprocity to keep them in line, cheaters outcompete cooperators. At first I was trying to understand what helps keep cooperation stable in human societies. But then I began learning about the biology behind cancer and the ways cancerous cells behave, and it became clear that lots of cancer cell activities looked like the breakdown of cooperation in a multicellular system. Cancer—which had seemed to me like a senseless disease, an organism destroying itself—started to make sense.

As I looked deeper, I discovered that cellular cheating manifests as cancer and cancerlike phenomena in many complex organisms, from humans to clams to cacti. Plants, for example, exhibit cancerlike protrusions called fasciations. One of the most striking examples is the crested cactus. Saguaro cacti can develop mutations in meristem cells (equivalent to stem cells in animals) on the growing tips of the plant. These lead to cell overproliferation and abnormal growths that fan out into crests. The fasciations can be quite beautiful, but like cancer in people, they can take a toll. Crested cacti often have disrupted flowering, which impairs reproduction, and are more vulnerable to disease and injury.

I realized that many of these breakdowns in cellular cooperation bore an uncanny resemblance to the "hallmarks of cancer," a framework developed by cancer biologists to describe general tendencies of malignancies. In addition to things such as excess proliferation, invasion of other tissues is one of the hallmarks of cancer, and an evolutionary approach suggests that invasion might be a consequence of cellular cheating. When cancer cells overuse resources in their local environments—producing enzymes that digest nearby tissue, for instance—the process often destroys their normal cellular surroundings. We know from ecology that organisms that deplete resources in their environments are under greater pressure to evolve the ability to move via "dispersal evolution."

Cancer cells respond to this same pressure to go mobile. I created a model of cancer that showed that higher rates of cellular resource consumption led to the evolution of cells that had a greater propensity to move, a development my colleagues and I reported in 2012 in *Cancer Prevention Research*. Our conclusion suggested that overuse of resources by cancer cells may be one of the pressures that drives cancer to metastasize, or spread. Even before invasion of other tissues happens, degradation of resources may push cancer cells to evolve the ability to move inside tumors.

This ecological and evolutionary perspective highlights new ways of identifying cancerous cells, beyond the typical hallmarks such as excessive replication. In 2017 biologist Carlo Maley and I, along with other colleagues at Arizona State, noted in *Nature Reviews Cancer* that scientists can look for cells that are not properly regulating other aspects of their behavior. These features include cells that are consuming resources too quickly or producing proteins and enzymes that damage the environment around them.

Catching Cheaters

The cooperation inside a multicellular body is not just about cells holding back from excessive activity. It is also about other cells working to detect and suppress cheating when it arises. Bodies have evolved ways of doing this. For instance, cells normally can replicate only with "permission" from their neighbors, which trigger the release of growth signals. And if any cells depart from the proper multicellular script, they are targeted for destruction by their cellular neighbors or the immune system.

Cancer cells also cheat detectors in their own genetic code. One such sentinel is the cancer-suppressor gene *TP53*. It codes for a protein called *p53* that plays a central role in many aspects of cellular control, from halting the cell cycle and initiating DNA repair to triggering apoptosis (controlled cell death) if a cell is too damaged. Other genes in our police force include *BRCA*, a crucial DNA-repair gene; when mutated and unable to perform its normal function, *BRCA* increases the risk of breast, ovarian and prostate cancer.

Genes in the *TP53* family (others include *TP63* and *TP73*, both of which help to maintain the integrity of the genome) evolved very early in multicellular organisms, first appearing in primitive creatures such as sea anemones, and offered enough of a survival advantage to subsequently spread widely across the tree of multicellular life. In 2019 Anna Trigos of the Peter MacCallum Cancer Center in

Australia and her colleagues reported that common mutations in cancer overwhelmingly affect signaling pathways that involve genes such as *TP53*. Furthermore, they found that there was a loss of communication between these genetic regulatory systems that evolved even before the evolution of multicellularity and those that evolved to keep these more selfish cellular behaviors under control during the transition to multicellularity. The scientists figured out the age of the genes using a technique called phylostratigraphy, which compares features of genes of existing organisms to determine a likely common ancestor, ultimately showing where and when in the evolutionary tree of life these genes emerged. They then looked at the mutated genes in tumors from more than 9,000 patients, finding that the genes that help to regulate multicellular cooperation were often compromised.

How do genes such as *TP53* spot cheating? They appear to function as information collectors about cellular activity. For example, signals about an increased number of mutations in a cell or heightened production of aberrant proteins flow to these genes from elsewhere in the cell and from other parts of the genome. Such signals most likely indicate that the cell is no longer cooperating properly with the multicellular body. And they trigger action by *TP53* and similar genes, which can halt the cell-replication cycle and initiate DNA repair. If these measures are insufficient, the genes induce cellular death to protect the organism from the potential threat that the cell might pose.

The two copies of *TP53* in humans come from our parents: one from our mother, one from our father. If one of these copies of *TP53* becomes mutated itself, this leads to a much higher overall cancer risk over a person's lifetime. People who have a rare condition called Li-Fraumeni syndrome inherit just one copy of *TP53*, which leaves them extremely susceptible to cancer.

Elephants, in contrast, have 40 copies of their version of *TP53*–it is called *EP53*–and several scientists, including myself, think this explains why the giant animals rarely get cancer. That absence of malignancy has been a long-standing oncological puzzle known as Peto's paradox. In 1977 Richard Peto, an epidemiologist at the University of Oxford, and his colleagues pointed out that larger (and longer-lived) organisms should get more cancer than smaller creatures because bigger ones have more cells and logically that should raise the chances of malignant mutations. Yet cancer risk and body size do not track, he noted. In a study published in 2017 and in ongoing work, our research group has found that this paradox exists throughout the animal kingdom. We created a large database of zoo and veterinary pathology records and learned that species that are larger and longer-lived have essentially the same rates of cancer as species that are smaller and shorter-lived; our continuing analysis has pointed to more instances of this pattern.

To us, this suggests that large and long-lived organisms have particularly good mechanisms for suppressing cellular cheating, such as those extra copies of *EP53*. Evolutionary geneticists have compared elephant genomes with reconstructed genomes of several related species—the woolly mammoth, for one—and found that as animals in this lineage got bigger, they kept adding more copies of *TP53*-like genes. This repeated occurrence suggests that the genes played an important role in the evolution of large body size. Big bodies helped the elephants and their kin survive predators, and the cancer-suppressor genes helped the elephants survive cheating cells in those big bodies.

This seems to be a pattern. Jumbo bodies have evolved many times in the history of life, both on the land and in the sea, and genes to check cheaters evolved with them. For instance, among cetaceans, the taxonomic group that includes dolphins and whales, a huge variation in body size exists. The humpback whale is approximately four times larger than the closely related common minke whale, and the orca can be 20 times larger than the closely related bottlenose dolphin. And the numbers of genes in the cellular-cooperation police force go up with body size in this group. Members of our research team, looking closely at the genomes of humpback whales, found duplications of genes involved in the process of apoptosis, when cells recognize they can no longer function properly and essentially kill themselves. Smaller cetaceans do not have as many copies of these genes. In the big whales, our group also found evidence of evolutionary selection for a number of genes involved in cancer suppression, such as cell-cycle checkpoint genes, cell-signaling genes and genes involved in proliferation. One of these genes, called *PRDM2*[T], regulates the expression of the cetacean version of *TP53*, which again shows the central role of that particular sequence of DNA.

Stopping cheating cells is not an easy task, because, in an ironic twist, malignant cells that stop cooperating with normal cells can start to cooperate with one another. That makes things even worse for healthy cells. For example, cancer cells can produce growth factors for one another. They can also help shield their fellow cheaters by producing molecules that help malignant cells cloak themselves, making it harder for immune cells to detect them. My group's computational models of cell populations in the body show that this kind of cancer cooperation can evolve and is more likely to happen when cancer cells interact with their genetic clones, events that often occur in tumors. This cooperation among rule breakers may drive their ability to successfully metastasize and invade other tissues. Cancer cells can move as a group, using electrical and chemical signaling, sometimes forming a long line of cells that works its way into other parts of the body. One study found that groups of tumor cells in the bloodstream are 23 to 50 times more likely to successfully generate metastases compared with individual cancer cells in the blood.

Improving Natural Detection

Cooperating cancer cells do seem like the stuff of nightmares, but understanding the role of cooperation among cells does let us think about new ways of stopping the cheaters, even when they band together. It may be possible, for example, to strengthen our natural cheating-detection systems. Some members of our research center are currently working on developing cancer treatments using elephants' abundant *EP53* genes. In test-tube experiments, they have already shown that splicing *EP53* into the genome can restore damaged *p53* functions in cells taken from human and dog osteosarcomas. The addition of *EP53* enhanced the usual apoptosis response that helps to protect the body from cancer cells. Treatments called immune system checkpoint blockades are another exciting area. These drugs block the ability of cancer cells to send misleading signals to immune cells–signals that hide their escalating cheating behavior–and they have shown some success in treating cancers such as melanoma.

Still another approach, called adaptive therapy, tries to weaken groups of cancerous cells by maintaining cells among them that are not so far gone. Instead of bombarding a tumor with heavy doses of chemotherapy–which ultimately favors the evolution of cells that resist the drugs, just as constantly spraying pesticides on crops leads to pesticide-resistant insects–oncologists have been trying a more restrained approach. They employ only enough chemotherapy to keep the tumor small. Allowing drug-sensitive cells to survive and compete for resources with drug-resistant cells can keep the latter population low. In early clinical trials with patients who had aggressive prostate cancer, this method kept tumors under control for at least 34 months, compared with the average for standard therapy of about 13 months. These tests are ongoing.

And because cooperation among cheaters–a warped honor among thieves–seems to be an important strategy among cancer cells, my colleagues and I have proposed blocking the molecules these cheaters pass back and forth as they signal one another to grow or develop new blood vessels to supply tumors. It would make it harder for cancer cells to work together. Given the ability of groups of cells to invade and metastasize more effectively, interfering with molecules that cancer cells use to stick to one another could be another future direction for therapies. Patients who have higher levels of some of these sticky proteins called plakoglobins have more metastases and lower survival rates, suggesting that the proteins are targets worth investigating.

The social lives of cancer cells within the body are much more complex than we could have anticipated. But our normal healthy cells are arguably even more sophisticated, and within them lie many weapons against cells gone rogue. We are not only bastions of cellular cooperation: each and every one of our cells contains within it a complex genetic network that can detect and respond to cheating. We are, after all, descended from a line of multicellular ancestors that suppressed cancer long enough to reproduce, and their offspring carried these traits onward.

In the big picture of the evolution of life, cellular cooperation has been wildly successful despite the persistence of cellular cheating. Cancer may break the body's rules, but we—along with whales and all other forms of multicellular life on this planet, honed by billions of years of natural selection—hold the tools for restoring peaceful coexistence.

About the Author

Athena Aktipis is an associate professor in the psychology department at Arizona State University and cooperation researcher. Aktipis is author of The Cheating Cell: How Evolution Helps Us Understand and Treat Cancer *(Princeton University Press, 2020) and host of the Zombified podcast.*

The Colon Cancer Conundrum

By Cassandra Willyard

In 2012, a few days after Katie Rich gave birth to her third child, she started experiencing sharp pains under her ribs. When she brought it up at her postpartum checkup, her doctor thought it might be Rich's gallbladder. Instead a sonogram revealed a spot the size of a dollar bill on her liver. It might be a bruise, her doctor told her. "You are 33 years old. Do not worry about this," she remembers him saying.

Rich did not have time to worry. Her oldest child was three, and her newborn was only eight weeks. "We were so overwhelmed with the three little kids," she says. But she did follow up. A biopsy revealed stage IV colon cancer. Rich got the call on a Friday and spent the weekend crying. "I was in total disbelief," she says.

The diagnosis made no sense to her. Nobody in her family had ever had colon cancer. Rich, an athlete, ran and played volleyball. She exercised through all of her pregnancies. She made sure to eat a healthy diet. And she was young. Colon cancer was not even on her radar.

Stories like Rich's are increasingly common. Even as colorectal cancer rates for older adults have declined, rates in younger people have started climbing. In 2010 adults younger than 50 accounted for 5 percent of colon cancers and 9 percent of rectal cancers. By 2020 those proportions had grown to 11 and 15 percent, respectively.

The underlying reasons for this rise remain a mystery, one that is proving increasingly frustrating for those in the field. Experts now recommend that the general public start screening at age 45 instead of 50, a stopgap measure that they hope will identify many of these cases. But it is hardly a perfect fix. The new guidelines will not catch the increasing number of cases in people younger than 45—people like Rich. And some worry that the influx of newly eligible adults could strain the system and divert resources toward younger, healthier people and away from older adults in underserved populations, who are already less likely to be screened.

If researchers could figure out who is at greatest risk, they could target those individuals for screening. The reality, however, is that the constellation of factors that are putting more younger people at risk has proved difficult to pin down.

Rising Rates

Cancer screening is designed to identify disease before someone develops symptoms. The rationale is simple: cancer is easier to treat when it is diagnosed early. And colorectal cancer screenings in particular can prevent cancer from ever taking hold. During a colonoscopy, doctors examine the colon with a flexible scope that allows them to take biopsies and remove precancerous polyps. These screenings have led to an overall decrease in colorectal cancer incidence and mortality—so much so that declines in the disease have often been touted as progress in the war on cancer.

But that progress masks a disturbing trend. In 2008 Rebecca Siegel was mired in data, deep in the latest update of a report by the American Cancer Society called "Cancer Facts and Figures." Siegel, a cancer epidemiologist with ACS, had run the numbers before. At the time the recommendation was that screening should begin at 50 for adults with no obvious risk factors. What would happen, she wondered, if someone broke down the numbers in a slightly different way and instead looked at incidence among people younger than 50?

To her surprise, that analysis showed that colorectal cancer rates were going up. Between 1992 and 2005 the overall incidence for people 20 to 49 years old increased 1.5 percent a year in men and 1.6 percent a year in women. (The rise was largely driven by rectal cancer, which rose 3.5 percent a year in men and 2.9 percent a year in women.) The numbers were even more stark when she broke them down by race: Per year, incidence had increased among white men by 2.0 percent and in white women by 2.2 percent. There was no statistically significant change in Hispanic women, but she found an increase in Hispanic men of 2.7 percent a year. The absolute risk for these younger people was small compared with the risk for older people, but Siegel found the trend troubling.

Declines in disease in the over-50 age groups had made it appear that colorectal cancer incidence was going down overall. But, Siegel says, "What's going on in the younger age groups is really masked."

Siegel published her results in 2009. "It got a little bit of attention," she says, but reactions were mixed. The consensus at the time was that screening should begin at 50. Rather than seeing Siegel's results as concerning, some argued that the increase was probably good news and attributed it to more young people being screened.

Siegel did not buy it. She points out that if the increase were the result of more screening, doctors would be catching more early-stage cancers and seeing declining mortality rates in this younger group. Instead, as she collected more data over the next eight years, she found more late-stage diagnoses and mortality rates that were climbing by about 1 percent a year.

In 2017, as evidence for rising rates piled up, the ACS's Guideline Development Group began to reassess its screening guidelines for colorectal cancer, tweaking models to incorporate increasing incidence among younger adults. When it lowered the age to 45, the benefits outweighed the harms. ACS updated its recommendations accordingly the following year.

The move "caused quite a stir," says Aasma Shaukat, a gastroenterologist at New York University's Grossman School of Medicine. At the time critics argued that colorectal cancer affects too few younger adults to warrant the change. Even today the risk of someone in their late 70s being diagnosed with colon cancer is about one in 500, whereas the risk for someone in their early 30s is about one in 17,500. And, the same critics said, there were not enough data to support such a shift in recommendations.

A Puzzle Unsolved

Today it is clear that the increase in early-onset colorectal cancer is real. In the 20-to-49 age group, rates climbed from about one in 12,000 in 1992 to one in 9,300 in 2015. "It's not just a blip," says Folasade P. May, a gastroenterologist at the University of California, Los Angeles. Some groups have been hit harder than others. The upward trend has been steepest among people who are white, Native American and Alaska Native.

Black people have had higher rates of colorectal cancer across all age groups for decades. "We still see young-onset colorectal cancer in Black individuals," May says, "but they were already having those high rates." Mortality rates are highest in these groups, too. But in adults younger than 50, she says, it is white men who are driving the increase. Twenty-five years ago Black people between 20 and 49 years old had a 40 percent higher incidence of colorectal cancer than white people in the same age group. As of 2016, the two groups were the same: one in 7,000.

Exactly what factors are prompting this rise is still unknown, but they are apparently increasing with each generation. In the U.S., people born in the 1950s have the lowest incidence of colorectal cancer, and rates rise from there. Someone who is 41 today has a 47 percent higher risk of colorectal cancer than someone who was 41 in 1991—over those 30 years the rate increased from 10.6 to 15.6 people per 100,000. In other words, the risk goes up with every subsequent generation and travels with those individuals as they age, something known as a birth-cohort effect. Other wealthy countries are experiencing similar increases. Siegel and her colleagues looked at rates worldwide and found that during the most recent decade of available data, trends in eight other countries resembled those in the U.S., with incidence increasing among people younger than 50 and stable or decreasing in those 50 and older. Rates among younger adults declined in only three countries: Austria, Italy and Lithuania. Two of those, Austria and Italy, initiate colorectal cancer screening for average-risk adults in their 40s, the very group driving those declining rates.

Researchers are scrutinizing the usual suspects—obesity, sedentary lifestyle, smoking, alcohol, diets rich in red meat and processed foods. One study showed that diabetes might play a role. Another found a link to sugary drinks. But for Rich and many others, those explanations do not fit. Actor Chadwick Boseman, who died of colon cancer last year at age 43, "was not obese. He was not sedentary," says Kimmie Ng, director of the Young-Onset Colorectal Cancer Center at the Dana-Farber Cancer Institute in Boston. "And that is reflective of so many of the young patients we see in our center."

Some researchers speculate that human papillomavirus (HPV), the cause of most anal cancers, may explain some of the rise in colorectal cancers in younger adults. That would mean that the vaccines that prevent other HPV-caused cancers might be protective. But most research to date has been unable to conclusively make the connection, and more research is needed to confirm or rule out the link.

Because the birth-cohort effect in cancer suggests that exposures early in life, during childhood or young adulthood, may be crucial, some have begun looking closely at changes to the microbiome. "We know that diet and lifestyle significantly shape our microbiome. They also significantly shape our immune system, which we need to fight off the development of cancer. And so we are hypothesizing that it's a complex interplay among the microbiome, diet, lifestyle and your immune system," Ng says.

Several case-control studies suggest that antibiotic use may be partly to blame. These medications can have a profound impact on the gut microbiome, potentially tweaking it in ways that foster carcinogenesis. And prescriptions for broad-spectrum antibiotics nearly tripled from 1980 to 1992. One study presented at the 2021 European Society for Medical Oncology World Congress on Gastrointestinal Cancer found that antibiotic use was associated with an increased risk of both early- and late-onset colon cancer.

Another potential explanation that some are exploring is gestational influence. Caitlin Murphy, an epidemiologist at the University of Texas Health Science Center at Houston, and her colleagues have been studying the effect of prenatal exposures on colorectal cancer risk. In a cohort of about 14,500 mothers and their children, maternal obesity increased a child's future risk of colorectal cancer. High weight gain during pregnancy also contributed to the child's risk.

That might be one piece of the puzzle, Murphy says, but it is certainly not the only one. "When I first started working in this area, I was kind of convinced that there was this smoking gun," she says. "The more I get into it, the more I realize that's just not true." Figuring out how the pieces fit together and who is most at risk will be essential for screening to be used to best effect.

Screening Debate

There is a growing consensus that the benefits of starting colon cancer screening at age 45 may outweigh potential harms. The American College of Gastroenterology, the National Comprehensive Cancer Network and now the U.S. Preventive Services Task Force have all endorsed the new lowered screening age. The U.S. Multi-Society Task Force on Colorectal Cancer, which is in the process of updating its guidelines, has also adopted the lower age for average-risk adults. (Those with a family history are advised to start screening even earlier.)

Lowering the age to 45 "really does make sense," Ng says. Because half of early-onset colorectal cancer cases occur in patients in their 40s, she says, "we will catch a lot more cancer in that earlier stage." At least one study hints that this may be true and that colorectal cancer incidence among people in their 40s might be even higher than anyone thought. A paper published in 2020 in *JAMA Network Open* reports an odd jump in the number of cases at age 50 compared with age 49. "That's not because there is something biologically different between 49- and 50-year-olds," says Swati G. Patel, a gastroenterologist at the University of Colorado Anschutz Medical Center, who was not involved in the study. Rather it is because when people start getting screened, cancers they may have had for years are detected.

The new screening guidelines should help doctors catch some of these cancers. Most adults younger than 50 have never been screened for colorectal cancer and can be slow to seek medical attention. One study found that for patients older than 50, a month passed from the onset of their first symptom to treatment. But for those younger than 50, the median delay was 217 days. Because they were not in the screening group and did not interpret the symptom as a potential problem, they waited to seek care or, if they did consult doctors, their physicians sometimes attributed their symptoms to something else such as hemorrhoids or fistulas.

Some researchers see the move to 45 as premature. If you look at the results of the modeling, Shaukat says, "the risk-benefit ratio is very, very thin." Screening programs are costly, and colonoscopies are not without risk. Scopes can cause bleeding or even perforate the bowel, something that occurs in about one of every 2,500 procedures. Plus, colonoscopies almost always require sedation, which may have its own complications. Stool tests can yield false positives—rates as high as 13 percent—which induce anxiety and lead to unnecessary procedures.

Increased screening poses hazards not just to individuals but to the entire system. Lowering the screening age by five years means 21 million people are newly eligible for screening. Many clinics already have a hefty screening backlog after halting colonoscopies as COVID cases surged in the spring and fall of 2020. Even where the procedure was available, some opted to postpone out of fear of exposure to the virus.

Now gastroenterologists must find a way to accommodate both the COVID backlog and people in their late 40s. If all these new recruits immediately schedule colonoscopies, they could overwhelm the system and lead to longer wait times for older patients who might have a more acute need. And screening compliance is already below what it should be in the over-50 crowd. According to Murphy's research from 2018, about 50 percent of white and Black adults in their early 50s are up-to-date with screening, compared with only about 35 percent of Hispanic and 32 percent of Asian adults the same age. And, as Shaukat points out, the healthiest and wealthiest adults in their 40s—executives who run marathons and eat kale—may be the ones who come in for screening first.

There might be a way to strike a balance. At-home stool tests can also detect colorectal cancer, and Siegel believes they should be more widely adopted. One system using them is Kaiser Permanente Northern California, which mails patients annual fecal immunochemical tests–FITs for short–if they are not up-to-date with their screening. These tests detect blood in the stool, something that can be a sign of cancer or precancerous polyps. Only those with positive results need to follow up, typically with a colonoscopy. Since Kaiser launched the program in 2006, the percentage of eligible adults in their system who get screened has increased from 40 percent to more than 80 percent. The national screening rate, in contrast, is just under 69 percent. Even better, cases of colorectal cancer fell by 26 percent among Kaiser's patients, and deaths related to colorectal cancer dropped by 52 percent.

The Veterans Health Administration has adopted FITs, too. When the pandemic hit, VA hospitals stopped performing screening colonoscopies for veterans with an average risk of colorectal cancer and instead began offering them a home stool test.

Siegel wishes more doctors would offer their patients stool tests as an option. "You don't have to get a colonoscopy. You can have a test that's less invasive," she says. "The reduction in mortality from colorectal cancer is comparable for both."

A newer test, Cologuard, combines FIT with DNA markers indicative of cancer. But although a single Cologuard test can detect up to 92 percent of cancers, compared with the FIT's 74 percent, it is much more costly and yields more false positives. Because it is recommended every three years rather than annually, the difference in accuracy over time may be negligible.

Neither test will help adults not yet eligible to be screened. "The rate of rise is actually the steepest in people in their 20s and 30s," Ng says. Colon cancer incidence is increasing by 2 percent a year in people 20 to 29 years old, compared with 1.3 percent in those 40 to 49 years old. Rectal cancer incidence is rising by 3.2 and 2.3 percent a year in those same groups. That is why we must figure out why rates are increasing. If researchers can determine those most at risk, she says, "we can target them for early screening rather than lowering the age."

Rich does not know why she got colon cancer so young and tries not to dwell on it. After her weekend crying jag when she was diagnosed, "I never looked back," she says. She put her energy into the fight ahead. After eight rounds of chemotherapy and the loss of 30 percent of her colon and 70 percent of her liver, Rich has been free of cancer for more than eight years. In 2015 she and her husband had another baby, a girl they named Hope. The chance the cancer will come back is small, but Rich still has an implanted pump her doctors can use to send chemo directly to her liver if it does return. "It's basically an insurance plan," she says.

This article is part of "Innovations In: Cancer Early Detection," an editorially independent special report that was produced with financial support from Johnson & Johnson.

About the Author

Cassandra Willyard is a science journalist based in Madison, Wis.

How to Tell Whether a Cancer Is Caused by Plain Bad Luck

By Viviane Callier

Cancer results from a combination of spontaneous mutations that arise with age—just call it "bad luck"—and environmental exposures to carcinogens such as tobacco, ultraviolet light or viruses. But the question of the relative contribution of luck—compared with more explicit causes—has generated vigorous debate for years.

The distinction matters because of the implications for cancer prevention: If a cancer is mostly caused by toxic exposures, then public health efforts should focus on strategies to prevent those exposures. But if a cancer is mostly the result of random mutations, then little can be done to prevent it, and efforts might instead focus on early detection and treatment.

Now a team of researchers has addressed this ongoing controversy with a degree of mathematical exactitude. Biostatistician and evolutionary biologist Jeffrey Townsend of Yale School of Public Health, Vincent Cannataro of Emmanuel College and Jeffrey Mandell of Yale devised a method inspired by evolutionary models of natural selection in wild populations to quantify how much every so-called point mutation, or change to a single DNA letter, in a tumor contributes to driving its growth.

Inside a tumor, there are usually many genetic mutations, but only a small subset of them "drive" cancerous growth. The rest are harmless "passenger" mutations. Using previous knowledge about the specific mutational patterns caused by exposures to carcinogens such as tobacco smoke or UV light, the researchers could estimate what proportion of driving mutations were caused by carcinogens and what proportion arose from accidental alterations in DNA that occur during normal cell division.

In the study, appearing in *Molecular Biology and Evolution* on April 26, the researchers used this method to investigate the causes of point mutations in 24 major cancer types. For each type, they were able to estimate how many cancer-driving mutations were linked to "bad luck." Confirming epidemiological studies, they found that melanomas and lung, bladder and cervical cancers are largely attributable to exposure to carcinogens such as UV light, tobacco or human papillomavirus, whereas brain and spinal cord tumors called gliomas and prostate tumors called adenocarcinomas are mostly the result of intrinsic mutations that accumulate with age.

The study "is a step forward because it's allowing a better assessment of the particular contribution of the agent– smoking, UV, et cetera–toward the actual driving mutations," says James DeGregori, a cancer researcher at the University of Colorado School of Medicine, who was not involved with the study. "Let's say you have a lung cancer with five driver mutations–you can say, 'These three clearly have the smoking signature, so they were directly caused by the smoking.'"

"There have been a lot of sidetracks taken over the years," says cancer researcher and oncologist Rameen Beroukhim of the Dana-Farber Cancer Institute, who was not involved with the new study, because people assumed that frequently mutated genes in a given cancer type must be contributing to the development of the cancer–only to find out that those mutations were just passengers. It has been important to understand the signatures of different mutational processes, but therapeutically, what Beroukhim and his colleagues are interested in is the small subset of mutations that are causing the cancer to grow.

For this reason, it has been tricky to pin down the definitive causes of a given cancer. And until now, the discussion has focused on risk factors–estimated over population averages–that could have contributed to the development of a tumor. Townsend says his team's new approach can be used to pin down the proximate causes of the driving mutations in a given patient's tumor and thus provides a more precise answer to one of the most difficult questions that patients and doctors struggle with after a cancer diagnosis: "Why me?"

One caveat of the study is that the researchers focused only on mutations in single letters, or nucleotides, of DNA, not large rearrangements of chromosomes or increases in copies of a gene that frequently occur in cells as they become cancerous. The reason is that the researchers did not have a way to quantify the selective effect of those large mutations in their evolutionary models, although they are working on methods to address that problem now.

These large mutations are not negligible in cancer cell genomes: in some cancers, one out of every 10 million nucleotides undergoes a point mutation, but one of every three is involved in chromosomal rearrangements or increases in copy numbers, Beroukhim says. Still, it is unclear how much these big rearrangements contribute to cancer growth because they have yet to be quantified for individual cancers.

Townsend acknowledges that the findings are limited because they do not take into account these large changes in the genome. It is possible, he says, that the percentage of point mutations caused by environmental exposures, as opposed to intrinsic factors, is approximately the same for these other types of mutations, so the conclusions would largely be the same. But that hypothesis still must be confirmed. "We'll learn in the future, but this is our first way of doing it," Townsend says.

In addition, determining causality in cancer remains a complex task. If a cancer-driving mutation does not have the signature of a carcinogen exposure, that does not mean that the carcinogen did not contribute to the cancer; it means it did not contribute to that mutation, DeGregori points out. The environmental exposure may have been indirectly responsible for promoting the development of the cancer by changing the mutated cell's environment, he argues. For example, smoking changes the environment in a smoker's lung, so a mutated cell inside that lung would behave differently than the same cell in a healthy nonsmoker's lung. The environment of a cell will influence its behavior and its ability to proliferate.

Townsend agrees that this context is important: in the same way, obesity, exercise or alcohol consumption may not directly cause (or prevent) mutations, but these factors change the metabolic environment in the body and thereby alter the risk of cancer, too. Future work will need to incorporate this larger context. Future work will also extend to more cancer types as more cancer genomes are sequenced and become available.

Despite these limitations, this novel method could provide insights into the age-old problem of cancer resistance to treatment: Frequently, a tumor will initially respond to treatment but come back after some time. That is because many chemotherapies themselves are mutagenic. The hope is that the mutations will be more damaging to cancer cells, which often lack good DNA repair mechanisms, than to healthy cells. But some of those treatment-caused mutations may enable the tumor to evolve resistance to treatment. Townsend and his colleagues recently used their evolutionary model to pin down exactly which mutations caused by treatment in a given tumor are responsible for the resistance to that treatment–thus informing which combinations or sequences of treatments to use or avoid.

The method's ability to address what causes cancer at the level of individual patients–something that had not been possible before–means that it could be extremely useful in legal cases, the researchers say. For example, it is typically very difficult to prove that a cluster of cancer cases in a community was caused by exposure to pollution or a toxic waste site nearby. But using this method to look at the tumors of cancer patients could establish causal links between exposure and a specific patient's tumor, which could have implications for legal liability.

"If this would have been available back when the tobacco lawsuits were going on, this would have been an incredibly useful, to be able to say, 'Here's the signature of tobacco smoking on all of these patients' tumors; you can't say that this is just some side effect,'" Townsend says. "It's nice to have a direct link between the tumor itself and the mutagens that caused it."

About the Author

Viviane Callier is a freelance science writer based in North Bethesda, Md.

Section 2: Detecting Cancer

Experimental Blood Test Detects Cancer up to Four Years before Symptoms Appear

By Rachel Nuwer

For years scientists have sought to create the ultimate cancer-screening test–one that can reliably detect a malignancy early, before tumor cells spread and when treatments are more effective. A new method reported today in *Nature Communications* brings researchers a step closer to that goal. By using a blood test, the international team was able to diagnose cancer long before symptoms appeared in nearly all the people it tested who went on to develop cancer.

"What we showed is: up to four years before these people walk into the hospital, there are already signatures in their blood that show they have cancer," says Kun Zhang, a bioengineer at the University of California, San Diego, and a co-author of the study. "That's never been done before."

Past efforts to develop blood tests for cancer typically involved researchers collecting blood samples from people already diagnosed with the disease. They would then see if they could accurately detect malignant cells in those samples, usually by looking at genetic mutations, DNA methylation (chemical alterations to DNA) or specific blood proteins. "The best you can prove is whether your method is as good at detecting cancer as existing methods," Zhang says. "You can never prove it's better."

In contrast, Zhang and his colleagues began collecting samples from people before they had any signs that they had cancer. In 2007 the researchers began recruiting more than 123,000 healthy individuals in Taizhou, China, to undergo annual health checks–an effort that required building a specialized warehouse to store the more than 1.6 million samples they eventually accrued. Around 1,000 participants developed cancer over the next 10 years.

Zhang and his colleagues focused on developing a test for five of the most common types of cancer: stomach, esophageal, colorectal, lung and liver malignancies. The test they developed, called PanSeer, detects methylation patterns in which a chemical group is added to DNA to alter genetic activity. Past studies have shown that abnormal methylation can signal various types of cancer, including pancreatic and colon cancer.

The PanSeer test works by isolating DNA from a blood sample and measuring DNA methylation at 500 locations previously identified as having the greatest chance of signaling the presence of cancer. A machine-learning algorithm compiles the findings into a single score that indicates a person's likelihood of having the disease. The researchers tested blood samples from 191 participants who eventually developed cancer, paired with the same number of matching healthy individuals. They were able to detect cancer up to four years before symptoms appeared with roughly 90 percent accuracy and a 5 percent false-positive rate.

The new study "offers several interesting approaches in the quest for a blood-plasma-based cancer-screening test," says Colin Pritchard, a molecular pathologist at the University of Washington School of Medicine, who was not involved in the research. It will be important, though, for another research team to independently validate the findings in a different group of people before the test can be considered for clinical use, he says.

Usha Menon, a professor of gynecological cancer at University College London, who also did not participate in the study, observes that Zhang and his colleagues' method provides a robust, preliminary baseline test–an "essential first step" toward a commercial cancer-screening product. "The authors are not suggesting that they have a test that can be used clinically at this stage," she says. "They are clear that what they have is a robust preliminary demonstration of early detection of multiple cancer types four years prior to conventional diagnosis."

Most likely, such a test would first target high-risk populations, Menon says. And it would require devising a second panel of tests to enable clinicians to determine the specific cancer type and rule out false positives.

Zhang believes such a feature could be developed with more work, and he agrees that further studies are needed. Given the challenges in repeating an effort of this magnitude, a government-industry partnership, he says, would ideally undertake the follow-up research. An ideal test would target the most common cancers, as Zhang's study did, as well as the deadliest ones. "There are cancers where early detection can make a really big difference," he says. Pancreatic cancer, for example, is the next target Zhang and his colleagues are working on.

If and when cancer blood tests do become available, Pritchard warns, they probably will not be able to detect all cancers before they become symptomatic. "One cancer might have a very long lead time, where another is very short," he says. "Cancers that grow very quickly might not be detected even if someone is, for example, doing an annual screening." It's possible, too, that some types of malignancies may never be detected by blood tests because they do not produce a measurable signal in blood plasma.

"We are still a ways away from having an accurate blood-based 'pan-cancer' screening test. But it is not impossible to achieve," Pritchard says. "There are several large efforts underway, with some promise for the future."

About the Author

Rachel Nuwer is a freelance science journalist and author who regularly contributes to Scientific American, *the* New York Times *and* National Geographic, *among other publications. Follow Nuwer on Twitter @RachelNuwer.*

Taking Early Cancer Detection to the Next Level

By Joshua J. Ofman, Azra Raza

Early cancer detection can save lives, yet, cancer is predicted to become the world's number one killer because we are still diagnosing most cancers too late. In the United States, we currently screen for only five types of common cancers. The rest are only identified when signs or symptoms appear, often signifying advanced disease when outcomes are poor. We estimate that these five single cancer screening tests collectively detect only 16 percent of the 1.2 million cancers diagnosed each year in those aged 50–79 in the US.

Medical students are taught that when it comes to cancer screening, sensitivity of the test is what matters. A screening test needs to find cancers that are present. Here is the challenge. We spend $27 billion annually on screening tests that yield about nine million positive results. Of these, only 204,000 turn out to be real cancers, while 8.8 million end up being false positives. Many women with suspicious mammograms know this harrowing journey too well, subjected to months of additional diagnostic tests only to be eventually declared as cancer-free. In fact, the screening tests recommended for a 60-year-old female with a history of smoking (screening for breast, colon, cervical and lung cancers), yield a 43 percent likelihood of at least one false positive test. This high sensitivity but suboptimal specificity approach to cancer screening targets one cancer at a time, taking decades to be adopted in a form where benefits are maximized, harms are minimized and the effort is cost-effective.

The importance of striking a balance between highly accurate and sensitive testing and screening a large population became apparent in the case of COVID-19. It is time to adopt a similar population-based strategy for other public health issues, such as cancer.

Improving early cancer detection may be the only way to really put a dent in the cancer mortality curve; however, early cancer detection is suffering from a common ailment in medicine and public health: the streetlight effect. We are looking for five cancers "over here" under the streetlight where we have early detection tests, but about 70 percent of cancer deaths are occurring "over there," in the dark, where we aren't even looking. Some may assume that we aren't screening for these cancers because we don't have treatments, but a review of practice guidelines and the literature shows that nearly all early cancers have effective treatments, even if watchful waiting is recommended for some, such as nonaggressive early prostate cancers.

Patients don't get to choose which cancer they get. So, what if we transition away from screening for individual cancers, and start screening individuals for all possible cancers? What if we dramatically improved overall cancer detection? What if we shifted to tracking the cancer detection rate (CDR) in the population?

First, the CDR represents the overall number of cancers detected out of the overall number of expected cancers in the monitored population. It is a measure of the population yield of a screening program. In the U.S., for example, there will be about 1.2 million cases of cancer in adults in the age range of 50–79 this year; mammography is expected to detect 114,000 of those cancers, for a CDR of approximately 9 percent. Even when all five single-cancer screening tests are combined, the CDR is still only approximately 16 percent. While an enormous accomplishment, this alone will not bend the cancer mortality curve or address the public health crisis posed by cancer.

The genomic revolution provides an opportunity to rewrite this chapter, with a potentially happier ending. There are now a number of novel multi-cancer early detection (MCED) tests nearing commercial availability. These MCEDs use sophisticated technologies to find footprints of early cancers in readily accessible body substances like blood, urine, saliva or stool. Several novel tests in development are able to detect a variety of cancers, many of which are potentially lethal cancers with no recommended screening tests. Such tests should be used in concert with existing single cancer screening tests, during preventive care visits or routine blood tests, which approximately 70 percent of Americans aged 50–79 have at least annually. If everyone took an annual blood test in addition to current screening tests, it could detect 50 percent for all cancers—including the deadliest ones, like pancreatic, stomach and lung cancers, that have five-year survival rates of less than 50 percent.

Why is MCED such a profound, game-changing idea? Because it is simply not feasible to spend decades in developing and testing a new screening approach for each individual cancer. With increases in cancer detection rates coupled with low false-positive rates, the balance would shift towards greater benefit than harm to the population. Used alone, MCED tests may still miss some cancers, but some detection is better than no detection. From a public health perspective, a 50 percent CDR could lead to the early discovery of many cancers when potentially curative treatment is available.

Just as we track COVID-19 infection rates, detection rates and death rates, we need to embrace the CDR model and track our progress in early cancer detection. Utilizing genomic signatures to dramatically improve the CDR may just be one of the first population-level benefits directly attributable to the vast investments made in the human genome project.

About the Authors

Joshua J. Ofman, M.D., M.S.H.S., is the chief medical officer and head of external affairs at GRAIL, Inc.

Azra Raza, M.D., is the Chan Soon-Shiong Professor of Medicine and director of the Myelodysplastic Syndrome (MDS) Center at Columbia University in New York. She is the author of The First Cell: And the Human Costs of Pursuing Cancer to the Last.

The COVID Cancer Effect

By Usha Lee McFarling

As the novel coronavirus swept through Boston last March, Toni Choueiri was worried. He was concerned not only about the rapid rise in COVID infections but about the swift shutdown in cancer screenings.

In Boston—and around the nation—colonoscopy suites stood empty as patients refused to come in, terrified of setting foot in any hospital or clinic. Screening center schedules, once full of mammography appointments, cleared dramatically. Hospital corridors quieted; screening center workers were sent home. Hospital administrators struggled to find enough PPE to take care of urgent surgeries, and elective procedures fell to the wayside. As COVID cases surged frighteningly across the country, cancer detection seemed to be the last thing on anyone's mind.

Choueiri, who directs the Lank Center for Genitourinary Oncology at the Dana-Farber Cancer Institute, saw a steep drop in new consultations in the pandemic's early months. The veteran oncologist feared that the lack of screenings, which aim to detect cancer at its earliest stages, would lead to a tidal wave of missed diagnoses. He worried about tumors seeding, taking hold, growing and metastasizing without being detected. He envisioned a future with streams of patients who had cancers so advanced he could no longer cure them.

Driven by these concerns and a desire to know exactly how bad the problem was, Choueiri and his colleagues turned to the data. Their study, published in *JAMA Oncology* in January 2021, showed a steep drop in screening from March to June of 2020 in his health system, Massachusetts General Brigham. More than 60,000 patients are typically screened there for cancer in a three-month period; in the first three months of the pandemic, he says, fewer than 16,000 came in for tests. In those early days National Cancer Institute officials estimated the pandemic would result in 10,000 excess cancer deaths in breast and colon cancer alone over the coming decade.

Screenings for some cancers fell by 90 percent when COVID struck, making a postpandemic surge of cancer deaths seem a foregone conclusion. As the pandemic wore on, some cancer centers began to report a worrisome increase in advanced cancer diagnoses. But as more time passed and screenings resumed, the outlook grew less dire. COVID may prove to be a grand experiment assessing the import of cancer screening, and results are beginning to trickle in. But because both the disease and its epidemiology are so complex, those results may take years, or even decades, to become clear.

Skipped Screenings

One patient whose pandemic screening turned up early-stage breast cancer was Senator Amy Klobuchar of Minnesota. After delaying the procedure, she had a routine mammogram in February 2021. With surgery and radiation completed and a good prognosis in hand, Klobuchar is urging others not to put off their screenings. "I hope my experience is a reminder for everyone of the value of routine health checkups, exams and follow-through," she wrote in a recent blog post.

Cancer kills some 600,000 people in the U.S. every year. Screening tests such as Pap smears, mammograms, colonoscopies, lung scans and prostate-specific antigen tests clearly save lives: although rates vary by cancer type, five-year survival is consistently higher when the disease is caught in its early stages. Yet as the pandemic spread throughout the U.S. and the world, rates of those routine screenings fell precipitously. This was especially true for colonoscopies, the most invasive screening and an exam that many avoided even before the pandemic. Choueiri's health system usually performs more than 9,000 colonoscopies in any three-month period; in March, April and May of last year, there were just over 1,700 in total. Similar drop-offs were seen across the country, where in some cases up to 95 percent of colonoscopies were missed in the first months of the pandemic.

Screening rates synchronized with pandemic waves, bouncing back in the summer of 2020 before falling during subsequent surges. Those who never rescheduled may be up to two years behind. "Between the peaks, what we didn't see was sufficient recovery," says Karen E. Knudsen, chief executive officer of the American Cancer Society. "We've made progress getting people back in the door, but there's a large population that is underscreened. We don't know the impact of this yet, but it's definitely a problem."

One major issue, Knudsen says, is that people who miss screenings aren't always flagged for follow-up. And some tests, such as those for prostate cancer, are harder to track using medical records because of how they are coded. In fact, she says, determining how many people are overdue for screening is virtually impossible because of the diverse settings in which patients receive screenings and because there is no national infrastructure that tracks them in real time. "We don't know who didn't come back," Knudsen says.

According to a study published in *JAMA Oncology* in April, nearly 10 million people missed screenings for breast, colon and prostate cancer between March and May of 2020, but no one knows how many of those tests remain unscheduled. Those who missed screenings, Knudsen says, are likely to be people who haven't been screened before, because they either just became eligible during the pandemic or were already hesitant. "We can infer that hesitancy is only enhanced with COVID," Knudsen says.

Tracking Missing Patients

Coaxing overdue patients into a clinic is one of Rachel Issaka's primary concerns. Issaka, a gastroenterologist and assistant professor at the Fred Hutchinson Cancer Research Center and University of Washington, says it is critical that health systems track down these missing patients. A study she published in June found that hundreds of colonoscopies were canceled between March and May 2020, and more than half of those people had not yet returned. Of those who did, more than 5 percent had new cancers. That implies that around 5 percent of the people who haven't returned may also have cancer, she says, but won't know it. Similar scenarios are likely playing out at health systems across the country; a study that surveyed gastroenterology practices last year found that two thirds did not yet have a plan in place to follow up on missed appointments, although some have now begun this work in earnest.

Issaka is working diligently to contact and shepherd in her more skittish patients. One powerful tool is at-home detection tests for colon cancer. A low-cost fecal immunochemical test, or FIT, can detect blood or tumor DNA in stools and catch 70 percent of colon cancer cases. But a positive FIT result requires a follow-up colonoscopy, and scheduling that, Issaka says, remains challenging.

Telehealth has proved a surprisingly effective way to persuade overdue patients to visit the clinic. A study published in *JAMA Oncology* last spring examined the precipitous drop in breast, colon and prostate cancer screenings and found that telehealth patients were more likely to come in for exams. Patients who are concerned about in-person screenings can use telehealth appointments to talk with their primary care physicians about setting up a plan based on personal and familial risk factors, says the American Cancer Society's Knudsen. "Screening is knowledge. It's power," she says.

Although much communication in oncology, particularly of bad news, is best done in person, the pandemic has shown that telemedicine can play an important role in cancer care and should remain in place, says Choueiri, who is also a professor of medicine at Harvard Medical School. "It's helped a lot," he says. "We can stay in touch with patients, maybe even better than before."

The pandemic-imposed challenges to screening prompted the American Cancer Society to create tool kits explaining current screening guidelines in clear and simple language. It is also spreading the word that patient access to screening must be made easier. One way is to move screenings out of hospitals and into clinics and, when possible, even mobile vans. Another is to open up scheduling in off-hours. "Can you do screenings on Saturdays or in the evenings?" Knudsen asks. "Those turned out to be really popular times for mammography."

Uncertain Mortality Models

There is little doubt that the chaos ushered in by the pandemic will lead to more cancer deaths. But determining how many has been difficult: many cancers are slow-growing, their development can be complex, and factors such as treatment decisions play a big role in outcomes. To assess how missed screenings might affect cancer mortality rates, the National Cancer Institute turned to Oguzhan Alagoz, a professor of industrial and systems engineering at the University of Wisconsin–Madison whose research involves modeling both cancer epidemiology and infectious diseases.

"The question is really interesting because it's a combination of the two areas I work in," Alagoz says. His first estimates, unveiled in a widely read editorial published in *Science* in June by NCI director Normal E. Sharpless, showed that missed screenings might result in 5,000 additional deaths in breast cancer alone over the next decade. A separate group, looking at missed colon cancer screenings, predicted another 5,000 deaths.

When Alagoz produced his breast cancer estimates early in the pandemic, he thought the numbers might not be truly representative. So he worked to refine them, using better data with three powerful cancer models that incorporated numerous factors related to breast cancer–such as delayed screening, treatment effectiveness and long-term survival rates–and the nuanced ways they intersect to affect mortality over time. "Everyone can tell you what will happen immediately, but it's hard to say what's going to happen in five or 10 years," Alagoz says. "If there's a huge increase in smoking, you're not going to see more lung cancer right away. You're going to see that 10 or 15 years down the road."

After a more detailed analysis and after seeing screenings rebound from what he calls the "panic phase" of March and April 2020, Alagoz now says those early mortality numbers were far too high. In revised estimates, published in the *Journal of the National Cancer Estimate* last April, Alagoz and his colleagues suggested the pandemic could lead to 2,500 excess breast cancer deaths in the coming decade, half as many as they had first predicted. "The entire estimate was too pessimistic," he says. "Any individual death is sad, but if there is any silver lining, it's that this isn't as bad as we feared."

One reason death rates may be curbed, Choueiri says, is that oncologists did aggressive triage work to screen and treat patients who needed care most. His hospital system reported fewer missed cancer diagnoses than he expected, and he thinks this was because people at highest risk of cancer and those with palpable symptoms were most likely to be screened even during the pandemic's most dangerous peaks. "Screenings never stopped 100 percent," Choueiri says. "Who were the patients who continued to be screened? They were the highest, highest risk."

Some oncologists say this "risk stratification"–prioritizing screening, diagnosis and treatment for those most at risk or with obvious symptoms–should stay in place after the pandemic ends so treatment can be provided quickly to those who need it most.

COVID's Long Shadow

Understanding the pandemic's effects on cancer mortality is a complicated task because delayed screenings aren't the only factor involved. Increased alcohol consumption and reduced physical activity–behaviors common during long pandemic lockdowns–can increase cancer risk as well. But postponing an exam can be a major danger. In November 2020 Vincent Valenti, a retired screenwriter in Brooklyn, noticed his voice was hoarse. He attributed it to all the screaming he did on election night. But it persisted for weeks, and his girlfriend encouraged him to get it checked. Valenti, 71, refused. He wasn't going near a hospital or doctor until he was vaccinated. "You walked by hospitals, and there were all these morgue trucks parked outside," he says. "I knew something was wrong, but I wasn't going to go near a hospital." In February of this year, once he had received two doses of vaccine, he scheduled an appointment with an E.N.T. "She scoped me and jumped back," he says.

There was a tumor on his larynx, stage 3, that had almost reached his lymph nodes. It was a shock to both Valenti and his doctor. He wasn't considered high risk for laryngeal cancer because he doesn't drink heavily or smoke. After seven weeks of chemotherapy and radiation, Valenti says, there was no trace of the tumor, and a recent PET scan confirmed that the cancer did not metastasize. Valenti was told his cancer would likely have been caught at stage 2, or even stage 1, if he had gone in right away.

Research published in *JAMA Network Open* in August shows that Valenti is far from alone. The study reports that diagnoses of eight cancer types dropped nearly 30 percent during the first pandemic wave of 2020, rebounded somewhat during the summer and early fall, then fell by 20 percent during the pandemic's winter surges. Such consistently low numbers indicate that many cases will continue to be undiagnosed, the authors wrote.

Some programs have already reported an increase in the detection of cancers. Lung cancer, the nation's leading cause of cancer death, is of particular concern because it can be so aggressive. The University of Cincinnati's lung cancer screening program was closed for three months. When screening resumed, patients remained scarce, and no-shows were frequent. But among those who did come in, "we noticed we were seeing many more suspicious lung nodules than usual," says Robert Van Haren, a thoracic surgeon and assistant professor of surgery at the University of Cincinnati Medical Center, who analyzed the effect of the pandemic on cancer screenings. "Even small changes in the size of a lung cancer can be important for overall survival," he says. "That's the reason we're concerned about any delays or stoppages."

Whether the pandemic has already caused an increase in dire cancer prognoses more broadly is still an open question. Choueiri hasn't run the numbers and is not sure yet whether his practice is facing more advanced cancer diagnoses. So far the picture is worrisome to him, but it is less so than he originally feared.

This is largely because screening did rebound. If the pandemic was turning out to be a natural experiment on the toll of missed cancer screenings, thankfully it was one that ended earlier than expected. "Testing for many cancers, such as mammograms, has largely returned," says Choueiri, who has co-authored several studies tracking the pandemic's effect on cancer screening. "Why did it return to normal? Simply because the hospitals, and all of us, put measures into place to make this as safe as possible."

Deepening Health Disparities

But timely screening hasn't returned for everyone. Those looking at the data see disturbing gaps in the populations that are coming back and those that aren't, gaps that may be deepening racial and ethnic disparities in cancer care and mortality. At his health system, Choueiri says, fewer Black and Hispanic patients rescheduled mammograms from June to December 2020, even after screenings rebounded in other groups. Van Haren saw something similar in his Cincinnati clinics: more screening no-shows for patients at highest risk of lung cancer death, including those who were current smokers and those who were Black. "It's concerning," Choueiri says. "The pandemic may have accentuated racial disparities related to cancer screening that already existed."

Black people are already 40 percent more likely to die from colon cancer than other groups. Issaka fears those numbers could now grow worse. "Before the pandemic, African-Americans, Hispanics and Native Americans were not screening at high rates. With COVID, my concern was that these same populations that were hard hit by the pandemic wouldn't come for screening," she says. "I worry that five to 10 years from now, we're going to see patients in those groups presenting with advanced disease and higher mortality."

Because colon cancers are usually slow-growing, it's not too late to prevent these deaths. "We need to be very proactive," Issaka says. "We still have the opportunity to turn the tide."

One of the people working to do so is Kathy Briant, assistant director for the Fred Hutchinson Cancer Research Center's office of community outreach and engagement. Cancer-screening outreach was one of the pandemic's biggest casualties, particularly among racial, ethnic and low-income groups that have historically had lower access to screening tests and are far less likely to be up-to-date on cancer screening than white and high-income patients.

Briant has had to mothball the giant inflatable walk-through colon she used to send to events in tribal areas and gatherings of agricultural workers throughout Washington State. She has had to cancel all face-to-face meetings with at-risk older people, the same ones who are less likely to see her team's YouTube and Twitter messages. Hardest of all, she says, she had had to call off two years of health fairs that, prepandemic, provided information, cancer screenings, free health tests and colonoscopy scheduling.

The communities Briant works with are both the least likely to receive cancer screening and the hardest hit by COVID: minorities, frontline workers, and people who were losing jobs, struggling financially and dealing with SARS-CoV-2 infections. She learned relatively quickly that cancer screening was not a priority for many in these communities. There was fear of COVID, but there were other reasons, too: no time, no child care, a lack of health insurance or the inability to afford copays. In addition, their regular clinics often were too overwhelmed with COVID patients to provide wellness checks or screenings.

People had more immediate needs, such as finding transportation to vaccine appointments and someone to help if they had COVID. Briant's team pivoted from providing grants for cancer screening to helping in other ways. "Our agenda, yes, is cancer screenings, but we had to set that aside and listen to the community," she says. "They were thinking about survival. They were saying cancer screening is not important right now."

Issaka's research confirms what Briant was seeing. One study at her safety-net hospital found that patients already faced multiple obstacles to having a colonoscopy, including lack of transportation, no coordination among specialists to get tests scheduled, and difficulties with the bowel preparation needed for the test. The pandemic added more barriers, she says, such as requiring a negative COVID test before people could even walk through the door.

By responding to more immediate needs, Briant's team hoped to strengthen bonds and increase trust in communities they work with, something that will help them spread the cancer-screening message in the future. Sure enough, as restrictions loosened, she began fielding calls from community health leaders who wanted the inflatable colon sent over. The hypercontagious Delta variant has put those plans on hold—a colon is an enclosed space after all—so they have resorted to a video version until Briant can once again unleash her colon into the world.

Could We Be Overscreening?

Another piece of the cancer puzzle that the pandemic experiment may start to solve is a particularly contentious one. As cancer-screening programs continue to grow, an increasingly vocal group of physicians is arguing that too much screening might, at least for some people, be doing more harm than good.

These researchers contend that many patients, particularly those of advanced age, often receive more screening than they require. And those tests can result in more risk than benefit. "One of the biggest risks of cancer screening is the overdiagnosis of cancer tumors that are indolent and will never cause symptoms," says Jennifer Moss, an assistant professor in the department of family and community medicine at Pennsylvania State University, whose research has shown that 45 to 75 percent of older adults receive screening they do not need. She found that for colon, cervical, and breast cancers, a large percentage of patients were being screened after they had aged out of the recommended age limit. In all three cancers, overscreening was more common for people living in cities compared with those in rural areas.

Unnecessary screenings not only result in false positives but also come with other issues, including unnecessary medical procedures to remove cancers that might not cause harm and side effects, such as perforations during colonoscopies. Now they have the added threat of SARS-CoV-2 exposure. "Many older patients face greater risk from cancer screening than not screening," Moss says. "Especially in a time of COVID."

Moss wants to be clear that people who need screening, based on national guidelines and conversations with their physicians, should get it. And she believes that the pandemic will likely cause an increase in cancer deaths because of missed screenings. But she also thinks the past year and a half will yield important data on missed screenings that were not as consequential-data that could inform future guidelines. "The pandemic will definitely give us insight into when, and how often, and for whom, cancer screening is the most effective," she says.

Choueiri, for his part, is convinced that cancer screening is a singularly powerful tool that can catch cancers at their earliest and most treatable stages. "You don't want stage 1 to become stage 4," he says. "Or even stage 2."

These days his conviction is personal. Unlike many of his patients, who postponed their screenings during the pandemic, Choueiri did not. Because of the pandemic slowdowns, he had extra time on his hands. So, when he turned 45 last year, he took his doctor's advice and scheduled a routine colonoscopy. He didn't think it was urgent–he had no symptoms or family history of the disease. But his test turned up an unexpected precancerous polyp. Now, he says, he will not miss any future screenings.

This article is part of "Innovations In: Cancer Early Detection," an editorially independent special report that was produced with financial support from Johnson & Johnson.

About the Author

Usha Lee McFarling is a Pulitzer Prize–winning science and medical writer based in Los Angeles.

Most People at Risk for Lung Cancer Never Get Screened: Here's How to Fix That

By Simar Bajaj

In late 2014 then-40-year-old Katherine Benson was diagnosed with stage IV lung cancer and told she had less than a year to live. "She was stunned," says her father Rick Nolan, a former congressional representative of Minnesota. Benson had never smoked and was a young, healthy mother of four. "She's the last person you would expect to get something like this," Nolan says.

Lung cancer kills about 130,000 people in the U.S. every year—more than breast and colorectal cancer combined. But early detection makes a dramatic difference: if diagnosed in its localized stages, lung cancer has an almost 60 percent five-year survival rate. That number drops to 7 percent with late detection.

"Every day in the U.S., there's a jumbo jet full of people who are dying of lung cancer that could have had early detection," says Claudia Henschke, a professor of radiology at the Icahn School of Medicine at Mount Sinai in New York City. Indeed, most people at risk of developing lung cancer never get screened for it. Increasing outreach to at-risk groups and expanding eligibility could change that—and save lives.

Restrictive Guidelines and a Low Screening Rate

The most recent guidelines from the U.S. Preventive Services Task Force (USPSTF), an independent advisory panel, recommend annual lung cancer screening with a low-dose computed tomography (LDCT) scan. In two large randomized controlled trials, such screening reduced lung cancer mortality by 20 to 24 percent. But to qualify for screening, a person must be 50 to 80 years old, have a smoking history of at least 20 pack-years (a pack a day for 20 years, two packs a day for 10 years, and so on) and currently smoke or have quit within the past 15 years. These criteria are designed to identify patients who are at the highest risk and most likely to benefit from LDCT scans, according to the USPSTF's vice chair Michael Barry, a primary care physician at Massachusetts General Hospital. The guidelines were also updated last year from even more restrictive ones set in 2013—increasing the number of people eligible for lung cancer screening from 8.1 million to 14.5 million.

Yet Douglas Wood, chair of the department of surgery at the University of Washington and chair of the National Comprehensive Cancer Network's Lung Cancer Screening Panel, thinks the new guidelines are still too stringent. For one thing, he says, the age maximum is arbitrary—there is "no evidence that once you turn 80, the harms outweigh the benefits"—and overrides what should be a decision made between patients and providers.

Wood also disagrees with the USPSTF's third criterion, arguing that the risk from smoking does not follow a strict time cutoff. "If somebody stopped smoking 15 years ago, and they're worried about lung cancer, the only way they can be screened is to either start smoking again—or to lie," he says.

Barry dismisses the notion that the USPSTF guidelines could incentivize smoking. In revising these guidelines, "we did, in our simulation models, look at other [cutoff] points" for the maximum age and period of smoking cessation, he says, "and we came up with keeping with the [existing] recommendations." He points out that the major lung cancer screening trials did not include patients who quit smoking more than 15 years ago, so the USPSTF has followed their lead. "Other guideline groups have other rules of evidence than we do," he says. But in general, the various guidelines "are certainly more similar than they are different."

Nevertheless, some research suggests that the USPSTF's eligibility criteria—which help determine Medicare and private insurance coverage—leave out a lot of people. According to one estimate published this year in *JAMA Oncology*, 35 percent of all patients with lung cancer would be ineligible for screening under the new guidelines. For Black women with lung cancer, the figure is about 66 percent. Because of their lower rates of cigarette use, on average, Black Americans, Hispanic Americans and women all experience significant disparities in lung cancer screening eligibility. For example, according to a 2000 estimate, about half of women who get lung cancer worldwide have never smoked—and thus would never have met the screening criteria.

Barry says the updated 2021 USPSTF guidelines "preferentially increase the proportion of women, Black people and Hispanic people who are eligible for screening, so we've made a pretty big step." He also emphasizes that the organization cares deeply about equity in screening, adding, "We're always eager for more evidence to fine-tune the guidelines as we go forward."

A more immediate challenge for screening is that, even among those who are eligible, the actual number getting LDCT scans is very low. In fact, only about 5 percent of people who met the old USPSTF guidelines were screened for lung cancer in 2015. That's compared with screening rates of about 65 to 80 percent for colorectal, cervical and breast cancer in 2019.

There is no one reason for this gap, according to Jamie Studts, a professor of medical oncology at the University of Colorado Anschutz Medical Campus School of Medicine. Part of the low rate may be that determining lung cancer screening eligibility can be difficult for overworked primary care providers, unlike other cancer screenings that have simple age-based criteria. The gap may also be related to the stigma and fatalism around lung cancer, as patients often think they will be blamed for having the disease and will not survive anyway.

The key barrier, however, might be a lack of awareness among physicians and the public: nearly 70 percent of people don't know that lung cancer screening is available at all. Other cancer screenings have been around for 25 to 50 years, whereas the USPSTF only began recommending lung cancer screening nine years ago. It may simply take time to embed LDCT scans into the culture of health care.

Improving Awareness and Access

Patient advocates and researchers are hoping to speed up this embedding process, starting with renewed public awareness campaigns. Denise Lee, a 60-year-old retired public defender from California, knows their importance firsthand. Stuck in traffic on her way home from work, she saw a billboard telling her that lung cancer screening could save her life. Lee decided to bring it up with her doctor but was told she didn't qualify. A year later, after using an online quiz to determine that she was finally eligible, Lee followed up with her physician, got the LDCT scan and was diagnosed with Stage IB lung cancer. Now a four-year lung cancer survivor, she simply says, "A billboard saved my life."

Awareness campaigns don't need to be fancy, but they should be more regionally targeted and personalized, Studts says. Since 2014 he has headed the Kentucky LEADS Collaborative, where he works with a network of community partners to meet face-to-face with primary care providers, educate them about the lung cancer screening guidelines and address their concerns. Studts also highlights the importance of combining smoking cessation and lung cancer screening discussions, because both are critical for reducing mortality and because primary care providers already do the former. Beyond Kentucky, there may also be an opportunity to leverage this messaging combination in national "quit smoking" ads. But Studts emphasizes the need for an empathy-first approach given that antitobacco campaigns have historically helped increase lung cancer stigma.

Ashley Prosper, chief of cardiothoracic imaging at UCLA Health, thinks there's also a promising collaboration between lung cancer screening and other screening programs. In addition to doing outreach work to increase screening uptake in Black communities, Prosper works on the Mammosphere Project to assess eligibility for lung cancer screening among women who already receive mammograms. She calls this approach "opportunistic screening," a method in which the high adherence rates of one kind of test are employed in service of another.

Last year Hannah Hazard-Jenkins, a breast cancer surgeon and director of the West Virginia University (WVU) Cancer Institute, similarly launched LUCAS—a lung cancer screening unit operating out of a tractor trailer. This 18-wheeler traverses the back roads of Appalachia, following in the path of WVU's mobile mammography unit Bonnie's Bus, and provides lung cancer screening to those in the most rural parts of the state regardless of insurance status. After local providers evaluate patients' screening eligibility, LUCAS arrives to perform the LDCTs. The scans are read back at WVU, and patients are referred for follow-up care close to home. "We have to be more creative about bringing health care to people, as opposed to always forcing them to us," Hazard-Jenkins says.

Expanding Eligibility

Another way to facilitate screening might be to simply expand testing criteria, Henschke says. Since 2001 she has led an initiative to open lung cancer screening to anyone age 40 or older, regardless of smoking history, as part of a research protocol. "Clearly you are going to find more lung cancers in people who have a greater smoking history," she says, "but one quarter of people diagnosed each year with lung cancer are never smokers." Henschke doesn't want to deny these patients a lifesaving tool. Nolan, the former congressman, agrees with her and similarly wants lung cancer screening to be covered for everyone age 40 or above. He helped craft Katherine's Lung Cancer Early Detection and Survival Act of 2020 (named for his daughter) to make this a law. Although a revised version of the bill was introduced in Congress last year, it hasn't yet been voted on.

If passed, this act would represent a major shift from the USPSTF guidelines. Nolan says that it would open access to individuals who do not meet the age criteria but are still at high risk of lung cancer because of family history, exposure to the radioactive gas radon or other risk factors unrelated to smoking. "I think extending the screening criteria, like at Mount Sinai, is appropriate if it's done as part of a clinical trial," Wood says. He is more cautious about making this expansion a law, however. "Unfortunately, as much as I see patients every week that have never smoked and have lung cancer, it is still uncommon," Wood adds. "And there's a trade-off in terms of benefits and harms."

Balancing Risks and Benefits

Barry says potential harms include false-positive results that lead to anxiety and additional testing–and the overdiagnosis and treatment of small lung nodules that would never have become life-threatening. The radiation exposure from the scan itself can also increase cancer risk. Prosper acknowledges these considerations and the need to discuss them with patients. She notes, however, that radiation risk is minimal with the LDCT scan–equivalent to six months of natural background radiation–and that false-positive rates are declining. These rates were 22 percent for the baseline scan and 27 percent for follow-up scans in the 2011 National Lung Screening Trial but dropped to 5 to 13 percent with the Lung CT Screening Reporting and Data System (Lung-RADS), a classification tool that standardizes radiologists' reporting and follow-up recommendations.

Hazard-Jenkins acknowledges that overdiagnosis is indeed a significant problem in the case of breast cancer. But for lung cancer, she says, "at the moment, I'm not sure you could overscreen because we're so profoundly underscreening."

Ultimately, the stakes involved in lung cancer screening–and in getting it right–are immense. "Policy makers have to understand that lung cancer screening is currently the most significant missed opportunity to change cancer outcomes bar none," Studts says. Though experts disagree on the best ways to deploy LDCT scans, nearly all of them agree that the 5 percent screening rate is unacceptable.

A couple of hours before Benson died, Nolan told her, "I'm looking forward to being with you as soon as possible." She responded, "No Dad, not until you get my bill passed." Nolan says he's working on his daughter's dying wish to help save the hundreds of thousands of people in the U.S. who still die from lung cancer every year.

About the Author

Simar Bajaj is a student studying the history of science at Harvard University. He has previously written for TIME, The Washington Post, The Guardian, Smithsonian Magazine, *and* The New England Journal of Medicine. *Follow him on Twitter @SimarSBajaj.*

When Should You Get a Mammogram?

By Lauren J. Young

When it comes to detecting breast cancer, regular testing matters. But precisely how early and how often you should get screened isn't so straightforward. Medical guidance can seem bewilderingly inconsistent. Some agencies recommend annual checks from age 40 onward, for example, while others have said to wait until age 50. There is no "generalizable" age that can be applied to everyone, says Vivian Bea, section chief of breast surgical oncology at New York–Presbyterian Brooklyn Methodist Hospital.

"I think we need a more personalized approach for each individual in determining when they should actually start screening—not this bucketed start age," Bea says. "We're clearly missing people."

Not only have breast cancer rates been climbing in the past decade, but people are being diagnosed younger. And now several medical regulatory boards and organizations are saying that if you're age 40, it's time to get regular mammograms. Last month the U.S. Preventive Services Task Force (USPSTF), an independent group of clinicians and researchers, proposed that people ages 40 to 74 receive mammograms every two years—an update from previous guidelines that recommended starting at age 50 and left it up to the individual and their clinician to decide on screening as early as age 40. These recommendations apply to people assigned female at birth, including cisgender women, transgender men and nonbinary people. Task force members also noted data showing disproportionate rates of late-stage breast cancer diagnoses and death among people in certain racial and ethnic communities, especially Black women.

"We have new and more inclusive evidence that getting breast cancer screening starting at age 40, every other year, will save lives," says task force member John Wong, who helped draft the proposal and is a primary care clinician at Tufts Medical Center. "That will help women who are Black even more and reduce some of the health inequity."

Why Does Age Matter for Mammograms?

Generally, breast cancer is more likely to develop with age because the risk of genetic mutations increases, and the mutations become harder to repair. Natural shifts in hormones can also play a role. "Breast cancer is more likely to occur when we're older, but we do know a lot of people who are getting breast cancer in their 40s and younger," says Laurie Margolies, a radiologist and the director of breast imaging for the Mount Sinai Health System in New York City.

For its proposal, the USPSTF applied newer and more inclusive data to a comparative model that showed what the survival outcomes would be for average-risk 40-year-olds in the U.S. if they did or did not receive breast cancer screenings. "We say more inclusive because these data include more racially, ethnically diverse populations than the original randomized controlled trials done for breast cancer screening over roughly 20 or more years ago," Wong says. What the data showed was "more women than ever before in their 40s have been developing breast cancer."

Long-term data from the National Cancer Institute show that breast cancer rates increased 2.7 percent annually among women under the age of 50 between 2016 and 2019—compared with a 0.3 percent annual increase between 1994 and 2016. Getting tested is an important step in improving survival and avoiding invasive treatments, Margolies says. "If you detect cancer by screening, you're less likely to need a mastectomy, you're less likely to need chemotherapy, and you're less likely to need to have all the lymph nodes under your arm removed," she adds. "So it's so important."

Many medical organizations have already been guiding practitioners to screen people for breast cancer earlier than age 50. The American College of Radiology has been recommending mammograms as early as age 40 for average-risk women. The American Cancer Society says women between ages 40 and 44 should have the option to get mammograms and that screening should start for all women by age 45. "A large percentage, if not the majority, of physicians in the United States have been recommending [screening around age 40] to their patients," Margolies says. But she adds that some insurance companies, particularly those supplying government insurance plans, as well as some public health departments and legislators, often lean on the USPSTF's recommendations to guide practice and policy.

Most insurance plans cover mammogram screenings, but additional tests such as ultrasounds or magnetic resonance imaging (MRI) may vary by state or require insurance authorization. Wong says the task force recognizes that insurance coverage and screening costs are important–but he notes that these decisions are not under the task force's control and remain at the jurisdiction of payers, insurers and legislators.

How Do You Know if You're at High Risk for Breast Cancer?

Starting screening at 40 can "save more lives–assuming you're not at high risk," Margolies says.

Medical organizations such as the American College of Radiology, along with breast specialists such as Margolies and Bea, encourage people to receive a breast cancer risk assessment at age 25. Practitioners use a risk assessment tool, which is like a "calculator" that crunches a patient's medical, family and reproductive history. If the result is above a certain percentage, a person is deemed at high risk for breast cancer.

People at high risk "may need more than screening mammography. They may need to start earlier. They may need to have supplemental MRI or supplemental ultrasound," Margolies says. "So it's a complicated message."

Two-dimensional-image mammograms are the cornerstone of breast cancer screening tests. Additionally, three-dimensional mammograms, or digital breast tomosyntheses, use several x-ray images to create a more complete picture of the breast, Wong says. Additional screening technologies look at tissues differently. Ultrasound machines bounce acoustic waves off body tissues to create an image, and MRI involves injecting a dye that helps visualize tissues and blood vessels in greater detail. "If you did just the ultrasound, you would see some cancers that you wouldn't have found on the mammogram. And if you do MRI, that's going to find even more cancers," Margolies explains. "For our highest-risk women, we recommend MRI."

Two of the factors considered during risk assessments are prior chest radiation exposure between the ages of 10 and 30 and breast tissue density. Around menopause, usually between ages 45 and 55, breast tissue typically becomes less dense and more fatty. Cancerous tissues are easier to spot in fatty tissue, where they appear as white spots or shadows on a mammogram. Denser tissue, on the other hand, masks some cancers on a mammogram. And cancers are more likely to develop in dense tissue (experts are still trying to figure out why). Wong says younger women tend to have denser breasts; about 50 percent of women in their 40s and 40 percent of women in their 50s are considered to be in this category.

A practitioner will also ask whether first-degree family members (such as parents or siblings) or extended relatives (such as aunts, grandparents or cousins) have had any type of cancer. More specifically, people with a family history of mutations in the *BRCA1* and *BRCA2* genes–which are important in suppressing tumors and curbing abnormal cell growth–are at higher risk for breast cancer. Certain populations, such as Ashkenazi Jewish people and Black people, are known to have higher percentages of *BRCA* mutations.

"Black women are twice as likely to be diagnosed with triple-negative breast cancer," a fast-spreading, invasive cancer with few treatment options, Bea says. "Triple-negative breast cancer is linked to sub-Saharan and West African ancestry. That's within your genes."

According to a 2021 study in the journal *Cancer*, women in racial or ethnic minority groups are 127 percent more likely to die of breast cancer before age 50 than non-Hispanic white women. And research in 2019 found that Black women are also 42 percent more likely to die from breast cancer despite similar diagnosis rates and are more likely to be diagnosed with later stages of the disease. There are several reasons for these disparities, Bea says. On top of genetic and biological risk factors, Black women and other members of minority groups experience greater barriers to quality care. "Confusion leads to distrust, and systemic racism also leads to distrust," Bea says. "Distrust, period, in the health care system leads to poor outcomes. We have to really have a unified approach to care that is more personalized."

Bea also suggests that women who are uncomfortable or nervous about breast screenings or risk assessments go with a trusted friend or family member. "Every woman should be empowered to know what their risks are and should start risk assessment at the age of 25," Bea says. "It is absolutely imperative that whoever's performing these assessments is aware of the intricate details of breast cancer and breast cancer inequalities in the U.S."

The proposal from the USPSTF doesn't currently include specific guidance on whether employing different strategies or screening earlier than age 40 would be beneficial for Black women, members of other racial groups or women with dense breast tissue.

How Frequently Should People Get Screened?

While several medical organizations recommend annual mammograms, the USPSTF's proposal calls for average-risk women to get one every other year; the task force says there wasn't enough evidence to show a benefit to annual screening for those in their 40s. Some experts, such as Bea and Margolies, say screening every two years is not enough. Lowering the starting screening age to 40 is a good first step, Margolies says, but she adds that younger women are more likely to develop aggressive, fast-growing breast cancers. "Screening every other year does not make sense," Margolies says. "We're lowering the screening age according to the task force to catch those fast-growing, more aggressive cancers. People in their 40s need it every year. Otherwise you're missing that opportunity."

Bea expresses similar concern for her patients: "I'm not going to [subscribe] to waiting for two years to use a perfectly invented tool—that we know works to catch it at its earliest stage—because there wasn't sufficient evidence."

Getting mammograms too early or too frequently has brought up concerns about false positives and overdiagnosis. For instance, if you are receiving imaging twice as often, you increase the risk of getting a false positive and of a clinician ordering costlier additional testing such as ultrasounds or MRI scans or even biopsies. "You do perhaps detect a few more cases of cancer [through screening every year], but we were not clear that that resulted in a lot of benefits," Wong says. An incorrect diagnosis might also be "unsettling and anxiety-provoking," he says.

Experts such as Margolies feel that temporary discomfort shouldn't outweigh finding cancers more readily. "How can you possibly equate anxiety, whether it be a few minutes or a few days, to potentially dying of breast cancer? It doesn't seem to make sense," she says.

Wong emphasizes that the task force's recommendations are meant to be built upon and that the group is calling for more research to determine if additional screening after a normal mammogram might be helpful. The USPSTF is taking public comments on its recent proposal for mammogram screenings until June 6. Task force members also plan to continue monitoring national data and trends as that information becomes available. Ultimately, they hope to answer the big question on researchers and clinicians' minds: What is causing breast cancer rates to rise at younger ages than before?

"Our lifestyle, our weight, what's in the environment–I think all those are combining to lead to increased risk of breast cancer. But we don't know for sure," Margolies says. "We might eventually find that maybe 35 is right. Maybe 40 is too old. These are questions that we'll need to answer over the next decade or two."

About the Author

Lauren J. Young is an associate editor for health and medicine at Scientific American. *Follow her on Twitter @laurenjyoung617.*

Section 3: Cancer Prevention

Do Cellphones Cause Cancer? Probably, but It's Complicated

By Christopher J. Portier, Wendy L. Leonard

Before you trash your cellphones (or rather, responsibly recycle and dispose of them), a careful review of the data–and the real life human implications–is needed. Here are the facts:

The National Toxicology Program (NTP) just concluded a massive 2-year study investigating the potential health hazards of cellphone use on rats and mice–most notably including the specific radio frequencies and modulations (RF-EMF) currently used in our U.S. telecommunications industry.

The NTP have chosen to publish their preliminary findings in rats, rather than wait. This study found that cellphone exposure increases the incidence of malignant gliomas of the brain, i.e., brain cancer, and schwannomas (also called neuromas) of the heart in the male rats. While schwannomas are not cancers, they are tumors and can profoundly impact the protective sheathing of the peripheral nerves, which can lead to severe pain and disability.

The increases were small (3-4 percent over controls), but since these are rare tumors, the findings are still significant. What make these studies even more significant are the *findings of similar tumors in humans*.

Human Studies: Pre and Post 2010

In humans, there have been numerous case-control studies of cancer and exposure to RF-EMF. The case-control studies (studies that compare exposure to cellphones of people who have glioma (case) with those who don't (control)) conducted prior to 2010 were all negative–meaning, no increases in tumors were found. However, those findings could easily be due to a lack of sufficient time for cancers to develop, or perhaps the sample size was too small.

Three case-control studies conducted since 2010 have all been positive (an increase in gliomas were found) in the highest exposure groups. Two studies found that the tumors occurred on the same side as phone use. These studies are subject to *recall bias*–people were asked about their cellphone usage and those with the tumor could have exaggerated their usage.

One study had high *relative risks* (comparing an exposed group to a non-exposed group) that would suggest we should be seeing an increase in gliomas in the general population. This has been examined in several countries with mixed, and often controversial, results.

Cohort studies, which follow people who don't have tumors to see if cellphone use results increases cancer risk, have also been conducted; the results were all negative. One of these studies had serious exposure misclassification (i.e., many of the people listed as unexposed actually used cellphones), and the other studies suffered from short follow-up times.

After evaluating these data, an International Agency for Research on Cancer (IARC) working group concluded these data show limited evidence of a glioma increase in humans. This means an association exists, but the data is not sufficient to be able to say they were certain the cellphones were the cause.

There have also been several *case-control* studies that specifically examined the risk of developing acoustic neuromas (a schwannoma of the acoustic nerve). As with the gliomas, the earlier studies were all negative, and most of the studies since 2010 have shown a positive risk ratio in the highest exposure categories.

So, why is this NTP study a potential game changer?

Back to the Rats

The NTP study is a long-term cancer bioassay in a specific strain of rats. There have been other long-term cancer bioassays in rats, all of which have been negative. Here's the thing: In all of the previous studies, the length of exposure and/or the magnitude of exposure was much less than what was used in the NTP study. For example, one study used almost the same magnitude of exposure used by the NTP (1.5-4 Watts/kilogram), but only two hours per day (the NTP exposed the rats for 9 hours per day). Another used 21 hours per day of exposure, but with a magnitude 10 to 20 fold less than the NTP. Finally, some of these studies used different rat strains, and it's well known that different rat strains don't always respond the same way to environmental exposures.

The new NTP rodent study is not without its critics. For both the gliomas and the schwannomas, there were no tumors in the control (unexposed) animals. Critics argue this inflates the chances of a *false positive* finding (that a certain result seems to have occurred, but really didn't). However, 50% or more of the recent (historical) NTP control groups have resulted in no tumors; thus, it's not an unusual finding. The significant findings remain positive if you compare the exposed rats to the historical control data. Another criticism is that there were no positive findings in the female rats for either tumor–again suggesting this was a false positive finding. However, male and female rats having the same tumor increase in the same site only occurs about 65 percent of the time.

In our opinion, the exposure to RF-EMF caused the tumors seen in the male rats in the NTP study. With the positive case-control studies seen in humans and a similar positive finding in a well-conducted laboratory study in rats, the evidence that cellphones can cause cancer has strengthened.

Do we think cellphones cause cancer in humans? Probably. But proximity matters, as does duration, and level of exposure. Think of it this way: sitting around a campfire is a fine thing, but sitting in the flames yields a very different outcome.

Steps You Can Take

1. With mobile phones, distance is definitely your friend. Exposure decreases as an inverse function of distance

from the head to the second power. This means that if you double the distance between your head and the phone, exposure is four times less. If you put it on the table, maybe about 50 times the usual distance from your head, the exposure would be 2500 times less. Thus, using a wired headset (or the speakerphone) with the phone on the table would yield a huge reduction in exposure. Before you ask, studies on Bluetooth headsets have yet to be conducted.

2. Carrying your cellphone in your purse or backpack rather than in a pocket or close to your body will also greatly reduce exposure.
3. Modern cellphones don't always emit the same amount of RF-EMF when in use. The better the reception, the less exposure from the phone. So limiting the use of your cellphone in areas of poor reception would also reduce exposure.
4. Turn it off if you are not using it.
5. If you feel grave concern over this issue, then don't use a cellphone. You might also want to prevent or limit the amount of time your children use a cellphone–since they will have much longer exposure over their lifetime.

Bottom Line

Cellphones probably cause cancer if the exposure is close enough, long enough, and in sufficient magnitude. We don't yet know the risk for a given level of exposure in humans. We need more data in this area, not only for cellphones, but for Bluetooth devices, wifi and all the other RF-EMF devices out there. Until then, reduce your exposure whenever possible.

The views expressed are those of the author(s) and are not necessarily those of Scientific American.

About the Authors

Christopher J. Portier is the former Director of the National Center for Environmental Health at the Centers for Disease Control and Prevention and was directing the activities of the National Toxicology Program when the study on RF-EMF was started. He currently works for the Environmental Defense Fund on issues related to air pollution, climate change and human health.

Wendy Leonard, PhD, MPH, is an award-winning medical writer, scientist, and best-selling anatomy coloring book author. Her passion is public health education.

One More Pioneering Woman in Science You've Probably Never Heard of

By Ellen Elliott

It is a regrettable fact that science has historically undervalued the contributions of women. Elizabeth Stern is probably one of the most significant physician-scientists who worked at the interface of epidemiology and cancer in the mid-20th century, but it is unlikely you have ever heard her name. You won't read about Stern's research in medical textbooks, or find any symposiums or departments dedicated to her memory. But her groundbreaking research led the way to our modern understanding of the prevention, diagnosis and treatment of cervical cancer.

Elizabeth Stern was born September 19, 1915 in Cobalt, Ontario. She was the fifth of eight children born to George and Sarah Stern, who emigrated from Poland to escape growing antisemitism and political unrest in Eastern Europe. She graduated from the University of Toronto School of Medicine on June 8, 1939, at the age of 23. While at the University of Toronto she met Solomon Shankman, a doctoral student in chemistry, and they married in 1940. They soon immigrated to Los Angeles, California, where Stern completed residency training in pathology at Cedars of Lebanon and Good Samaritan Hospitals in 1946.

From 1950 to 1960 she served as the director of laboratories and research at the Los Angeles Cancer Detection Center. In 1961 Stern was hired by the University of California Los Angeles (U.C.L.A) School of Medicine as the chief of the Cytology Laboratory, and began her research lab in the Department of Pathology. In 1963 her laboratory was transferred to the U.C.L.A. School of Public Health. Stern's former colleague and distinguished cytopathology expert Dorothy Rosenthal commented that, "The Department of Pathology didn't want to keep [Stern] ... because the Chair did not want to fill a full-time faculty position with a cytopathologist."

Cytopathology refers to the diagnosis of disease at the cellular level. The first cytopathology tool widely used in the United States was the Pap smear test, which was adopted in the 1950s to screen patients for cervical cancer. The Pap test has helped reduce cervical cancer frequency and mortality by more than 70% compared to the 1950s. However, few physicians in the 1960s were interested in further research connecting cell shape and morphology to disease. As Rosenthal remarked, "The field of cytopathology at the time was fledgling. A lot of people in pathology, and medicine in general, looked at it as if it were witchcraft."

One of Stern's primary research interests was the role of dysplasia in the development of cervical cancer. Dysplasia is abnormal cell growth that is non-invasive to surrounding tissues, and often reverses back to normal epithelial morphology. In the 1950s and 1960s the early stages of cervical cancer were not well defined, and although dysplasia was noted in smear results, it wasn't considered a cause for concern. But what if dysplasia was indicative of something more serious? Stern hypothesized that these morphological abnormalities could be an early sign of cervical cancer development.

To investigate this question, Stern and her group organized long-term epidemiological studies, in one report collecting Pap test samples from over 10,000 women in Los Angeles County. They carefully documented results of patients at the beginning of the study, and again at follow-up tests performed over the course of the seven-year study. She found that patients diagnosed with dysplasia at the start of the study were at significantly higher risk for cervical cancer. Stern would go on to lead over a dozen epidemiological studies providing nearly irrefutable proof that dysplasia is an early marker of cervical cancer.

It's difficult to overstate how important this discovery was to the medical community, and how innovative her theory was at the time. Today dysplasia is identified during routine cervical cancer screenings using the Pap test, and patients are monitored closely for further progression to carcinoma. The idea that dysplasia could possibly be seen as a debatable risk factor for cancer is preposterous today, largely due to Stern's meticulous and groundbreaking research.

Of all of Stern's achievements, perhaps her most lasting legacy is in the modern technology of the Pap test. She collaborated with the Jet Propulsion Laboratory (JPL) and Rosenthal, then the head cytopathologist at U.C.L.A, to apply NASA computer imaging technology to Pap screening. Stern developed a liquid-based sampling system to isolate and enrich the cervical epithelium, and helped define cellular criteria for computer programs. The work she did at JPL revolutionized Pap screening for cervical cancer, and her liquid-based sampling technique is still used in hospitals, laboratories, and clinics around the world.

Stern was also interested in other risk factors related to cervical cancer development. By again combining epidemiological analysis with cytopathology, she found that the original high-dose estrogen birth control pill increased the rate of cervical cancer six-fold. She testified to FDA advisory committees about this risk, and her research was quoted in news articles at the time on the questionable safety of 1970s era birth control pills. Her efforts were essential in prompting drug companies to reformulate birth control pills to protect women's health.

One of the reasons Stern's work was so comprehensive was her persistence in finding and screening at-risk women. Few researchers succeeded in recruiting at-risk populations, or enrolling them in high enough numbers to have reliable results. Stern's group published some of the earliest studies documenting the difficulties of poor women accessing preventive medical care, and demonstrated that providing help, such as childcare or transportation, can increase life-saving care to high-risk populations.

Stern continued working on her research after she was diagnosed with stomach cancer, and was writing manuscripts until her death in August 1980. In remembering Stern, I see someone that served as a strong and inspiring role model for countless women scientists. Stern had a challenging start at U.C.L.A. Her daughter Janet Williamson recalls that, "As a woman it was a struggle ... the first year she worked at U.C.L.A. she was not paid a salary." Through her perseverance she changed the way doctors diagnose cervical cancer, and shaped the field of cytopathology for decades to come.

Stern was a true embodiment of women in science. One of my favorite memories of Stern is from Marilyn Winkleby, a renowned epidemiologist at Stanford University, who credits Stern's lab for starting her research career. "I remember her being alone in her office working on her science. That's the picture I have of her. Sitting right outside her busy basic science lab. But the door was always open; the door was never closed."

The views expressed are those of the author(s) and are not necessarily those of Scientific American.

About the Author

Ellen Elliott, Ph.D. is a postdoctoral fellow in Adam Williams' lab at The Jackson Laboratory for Genomic Medicine in Farmington, CT. She is a regular contributor on The Jackson Laboratory Blog, *where she writes about women in science and postdoc career development. You can follow Ellen on Twitter @EllenNichole.*

Pancreatic Cancer Vaccine Shows Promise in Small Initial Trial

By Tanya Lewis

Pancreatic cancer is one of the deadliest forms of cancer, with very few effective treatments. But messenger RNA (mRNA) vaccines—famous for their ability to prevent COVID—are starting to show some promise against the lethal cancer. In a recent early-stage trial, half of pancreatic cancer patients who received a personalized mRNA cancer vaccine after surgery did not have a recurrence of the tumor a year and a half later. The trial, which was described in a study published on Wednesday in *Nature*, was small—with just 16 patients—and it will need to be replicated in larger studies.

"I am very supportive of the findings," says Drew Weissman, director of vaccine research and director of the Institute for RNA Innovation at the University of Pennsylvania, who is a pioneer of mRNA vaccines but was not involved in the new paper. He adds that "it is not a definitive proof-for-use study. Larger studies are needed to determine effectiveness."

Pancreatic ductal adenocarcinoma, the most common type of pancreatic cancer, has a mortality rate of 88 percent. It is the third leading cause of death from cancer in the U.S. and is becoming more common. Surgery is the main form of treatment, but the cancer has a 90 percent recurrence rate at seven to nine months. Chemotherapy is only partially effective at delaying recurrence. Other treatments, such as immunotherapy, are mostly ineffective.

Pancreatic cancer often goes undetected until its later stages, when it is harder to treat. One reason it is so sneaky is that it generates relatively few of a type of surface proteins, called neoantigens, that mark it as foreign and trigger an immune response. Scientists had noticed that people who survived pancreatic cancer had a stronger response to these neoantigens from T cells, a type of immune cell.

In the new study, Vinod Balachandran, an assistant attending surgeon at Memorial Sloan Kettering Cancer Center in New York City, and his colleagues targeted pancreatic cancer patients' own tumor neoantigens using mRNA technology–the same technology used to create the remarkably successful COVID vaccines. The experimental vaccines used by Balachandran and his colleagues were produced by BioNTech, a company that developed one of the COVID vaccines with Pfizer. The researchers vaccinated a total of 16 patients. After surgically removing the tumors, they treated the patients with mRNA vaccines tailored to each person's specific cancer, as well as an adjuvant, a substance that increases the effects of vaccines. Fifteen of the participants were also treated with chemotherapy.

Eight of the 16 patients generated a strong T cell response to the vaccines. At a median follow-up time of 18 months after the treatment, these individuals had longer survival, without a recurrence of their cancer.

The study was small and involved only white patients. And the therapy–which is expensive–does not work for everyone with pancreatic cancer. Nevertheless, experts say it is a promising development for a disease with such limited treatment options.

About the Author

Tanya Lewis is a senior editor covering health and medicine for Scientific American. *Follow her on Twitter @tanyalewis314.*

Having Their Fallopian Tubes Removed Will Spare a Large Number of Women from Ovarian Cancer

By Joseph V. Sakran, Kara Long Roche, Rebecca Stone

By the time someone has symptoms of ovarian cancer, it is usually in an advanced state. Treatment is extraordinarily difficult, and, sadly, most people will die. One in 78 women will develop ovarian cancer, and more than 230,000 women in the U.S. are currently affected. Of these, approximately 80 percent have no family history of ovarian cancer and no indication that they were at risk for developing it.

In addition to the lack of early symptoms, late stage diagnosis occurs because there is no effective way to screen for or diagnose ovarian cancer in its earliest forms. A recent study of hundreds of thousands of women showed that screening with ultrasounds and blood testing did not save as many lives as hoped. In fact, ineffective screening leading to false reassurance (via a false negative result) is a serious concern even in high-risk patients.

Despite the name "ovarian cancer," scientific discoveries from the last 20 years point to the fallopian tubes (two thin tubes that allow eggs to travel from the ovaries to the uterus) as the site of origin for the most common and most lethal form of ovarian cancer, high-grade serous carcinoma. Researchers found that cells lining the fallopian tubes are particularly prone to mutations in a cancer-suppressing gene called *p53*. These mutations allow for uncontrolled multiplication of cancerous cells and their spread throughout the body. In studying *p53* mutations in ovarian cancer, scientists traced them back to tiny precancers in the fallopian tubes.

With most ovarian cancers originating in the fallopian tube, researchers decided to investigate whether people whose fallopian tubes have been removed, which is done to remove an ectopic pregnancy, treat inflammatory processes in the fallopian tube and sometimes as a form of birth control, would have a reduced risk of developing ovarian cancer. Large epidemiologic studies show this to be the case, and it has been eye-opening for physicians like us. Given the seemingly insurmountable challenge of developing a screening test, clinicians are beginning to offer people who have completed childbearing and who are already undergoing planned surgeries the option of removing their fallopian tubes in order to prevent ovarian cancer. This strategy, called "opportunistic salpingectomy," is safe–and early data suggest it could reduce the risk of ovarian cancer by at least 65 percent. And as part of another gynecologic surgery, the preventative removal of fallopian tubes is supported by the American College of Obstetricians and Gynecologists and many professional societies worldwide.

Removing a person's fallopian tubes may sound like a radical idea, especially because elective procedures do carry risk, but in the U.S. alone more than one million women undergo hysterectomies or tubal ligations every year, which are often considered elective as well. A simple change in surgical technique–removing the fallopian tubes with the uterus during hysterectomy, and removing instead of "tying" the tubes for those opting surgical contraception –would add ovarian cancer prevention to two of the most common gynecologic procedures without the need for a separate medical intervention. This is a move we, as surgeons, believe is in the best interests of our patients.

For the time being, surgery is simply the best possible option to reduce ovarian cancer risk. While ultrasound and other pelvic imaging techniques are useful for visualizing the uterus and ovaries, they cannot reliably show us the fallopian tubes. Furthermore, cancer cells from the fallopian tubes likely spread while they are still microscopic. Technology that can both "see" the tube and identify microscopic precancers would be needed for effective screening.

It has been similarly difficult to find a biomarker for early disease. Known biomarkers are detectable in the bloodstream usually only after cancer has advanced well beyond the fallopian tubes and the adjoining ovaries. Since early disease progression occurs by direct spread of microscopic cells from the fallopian tubes and onto the surfaces of organs and tissues in the abdominal cavity instead of through the blood, testing for blood biomarkers may never prove useful.

Unlike removing the ovaries, which causes menopause, removal of the fallopian tubes has no known negative health consequence after child bearing is complete, and it adds nominal risk and time to the performance and recovery from the original surgical procedure. Salpingectomy during hysterectomy and in lieu of tubal ligation for surgical contraception was incorporated into routine practice in British Columbia more than 10 years ago. Researchers recently published preliminary data showing that this practice results in decreased incidence of ovarian cancer in the general population. The possibility that we could reduce the number of people affected by this lethal cancer with a change in surgical practice that has no lasting consequences after the completion of childbearing is a game changer. Extending this option to nongynecologic surgery would exponentially increase the number of people with access to the surgical prevention of ovarian cancer, and is the capstone of ongoing implementation research.

It's important that people have greater agency over their health, especially when it comes to preventing a cancer for which we have neither adequate screening nor a dependable cure. Work is underway to ensure that all patients desiring surgical contraception or undergoing hysterectomy are offered an opportunistic salpingectomy. In addition, efforts to scale this beyond gynecological procedures to operations like gallbladder surgery, hernia repair, and others are mounting. Saving lives from ovarian cancer can become a reality in our lifetimes if we offer the opportunity of fallopian tube removal to the hundreds of thousands of patients undergoing abdominal operations every year in the U.S.

This is an opinion and analysis article, and the views expressed by the author or authors are not necessarily those of Scientific American.

About the Authors

Joseph V. Sakran is an associate professor of surgery and nursing, and vice chair of clinical operations, at the Johns Hopkins Hospital. He holds M.D., M.P.H.

and M.P.A. degrees and is a fellow of the American College of Surgeons. Follow Sakran on Twitter @JosephSakran.

Kara Long Roche is an associate attending and member of the Section for Ovarian Cancer Surgery in the Department of Surgery, Gynecology Service at Memorial Sloan Kettering Cancer Center. She holds an M.D. and an M.Sc. and is a fellow of the American College of Obstretrics and Gynecologists. Follow Long Roche on Twitter @KaraLongRoche.

Rebecca Stone is associate professor and director of gynecologic oncology at the Johns Hopkins Hospital. She holds an M.D. and an M.S. and is a fellow of the American College of Obstretricians and Gynecologists.

Adjusting Your Body Clock May Stave Off Cancer

By Lydia Denworth

I usually get up by 7 A.M. and am in bed by 10 P.M. I tend to eat meals at the same times of day, too. This may sound a little dull, but it's essential for my productivity. It's also a schedule that rarely disrupts my body clock. And a steady clock, it turns out, just might help me and many other people avoid cancer and some other diseases, according to new research.

What I call a body clock really means circadian rhythms, from the Latin for "about" and "day." These are the body's internal biological pacemakers, physiological fluctuations that help us adjust to the phases of a 24-hour day by synchronizing with environmental cues such as light, dark, temperature and food intake. These rhythms affect sleeping and waking, feeding and fasting, endocrine cycles, immune function, and cell growth.

For some time now epidemiological studies of night-shift workers have linked disruptions in circadian rhythms to cancer and other diseases. Much of the evidence concerned breast cancer and to a lesser extent prostate cancer. Duration of shift work made a difference—nurses who worked night shifts for up to 30 years were at moderately increased risk for breast cancer compared with those who did shorter stints, and those who worked such shifts for more than 30 years had the highest risk. In 2019 the World Health Organization reaffirmed and updated a research statement from the agency showing that shift work is a probable carcinogen.

Now there is even more evidence involving other types of malignancies, including liver, lung and colorectal cancers, from a spate of new studies. "We're starting to understand the reasons these things happen," says Selma Masri, a circadian biologist at the University of California, Irvine, who has shown how circadian disruption pushes colon cancer progression by interfering with the way certain genes are expressed.

The cancer connection comes about through several mechanisms. Circadian disruption affects metabolic pathways, the chemical reactions that produce energy in the body. It tampers with immune function. It also compromises the fidelity of DNA repair in cells. Adult human cells divide every 18 to 24 hours, and one function of the circadian clock is to tell cells to do that at night to avoid DNA damage from sunlight. "When the clock gets disrupted, cells don't know when to divide," says circadian biologist Satchidananda Panda of the Salk Institute for Biological Studies. "They can divide faster and become a tumor."

Circadian disruption doesn't only occur in shift workers. It happens when we consistently don't get a good night's sleep–scientists say this can mean waking up for two or three hours between 10 P.M. and 5 A.M. at least once a week. Wakeful episodes can be caused by jet lag, staying out late, or looking at blue-light-emitting phone screens–which mimic daylight–at night. When and what we eat also cues our rhythms, just as light and dark do, so add snacking at midnight to the list of things to avoid.

The growing understanding of circadian rhythms also could offer help through what's known as chronotherapy. Certain chemotherapy treatments, for example, are more effective when given in accordance with a patient's rhythms. Now researchers are exploring differences in the timing of radiation therapy. Drugs that bolster natural rhythms are also under investigation.

Shift work is critical and not going away, says Katja Lamia, a circadian biologist at Scripps Research, but there might be ways of reducing its toll on the body. Her research suggests that subtle increases in body temperature might be an important factor in circadian disruption. If that turns out to be right, Lamia says, "we can use noninvasive monitoring of body temperature in shift workers to evaluate who's at risk and take a personalized scheduling approach."

For those who don't work at night, changing some routines might be enough. A good night's sleep should be a priority. Eating habits can also play a role. Panda and his colleagues are investigating a practice known as time restricted eating (TRE) or intermittent fasting. That might mean delaying breakfast by an hour or two until cortisol levels drop and eating dinner at least three hours before your habitual bedtime. In a 12-week study of firefighters, TRE benefited their metabolic health and improved their sleep. In mice, it has been shown to reduce the risk of cancer or to slow the growth of tumors.

Maybe, Panda says, respecting our circadian rhythms can help protect our time-sensitive bodies.

This is an opinion and analysis article, and the views expressed by the author or authors are not necessarily those of Scientific American.

About the Author

Lydia Denworth is an award-winning science journalist and contributing editor for Scientific American. She is author of Friendship: The Evolution, Biology, and Extraordinary Power of Life's Fundamental Bond *(W. W. Norton, 2020) and several other books of popular science.*

Section 4: Treating Cancer

Scientists Tackle Lethal Childhood Brain Cancer

By Esther Landhuis

Nine years ago on a Monday afternoon, Sandra Smith, a pastor's wife and mother of three in DeWitt, Mich., learned she had an aggressive form of breast cancer. The real bad news, however, would hit the family later that week.

At first they thought their youngest, six-year-old Andrew, was just battling the flu. Then he started vomiting. He'd also developed a facial droop, and his gait seemed off. Smith remembers wondering if they were "making a big deal out of nothing," even as they rushed to the emergency room.

Nothing could be further from the truth. An MRI scan revealed a large area of swelling in Andrew's brain stem—clear evidence of a fatal childhood cancer that typically strikes between the ages of four and 10 and kills most within a year of diagnosis. Unlike the cells dividing uncontrollably in Smith's breast, her son's cancer, called diffuse intrinsic pontine glioma (DIPG), could not be fought with surgery or conventional chemotherapy. In DIPG the malignant cells entwine with normal brain tissue in a region that controls critical functions such as breathing and heart rate, making it impossible for a surgeon to remove. In more than 200 drug trials nothing has worked better than radiation therapy, which itself can only extend life a few short months in kids with DIPG. Andrew outlived the "typical" DIPG patient by surviving just over two years after his diagnosis, passing away at the end of 2009.

DIPG accounts for about 10 percent of childhood brain and spinal cord tumors. It is the second-most common pediatric brain tumor and the leading cause of cancer death in kids. Treatment options and survival rate for DIPG have not changed in 40 years—a predicament that likely helped nudge brain cancer past leukemia as the deadliest childhood malignancy in the nation, according to a recent report from the U.S. Centers for Disease Control and Prevention.

Today, however, the outlook for DIPG and other childhood brain cancers looks more promising, thanks to a surge of new research made possible by advances in gene-sequencing methods and tumor tissue donations from families who have lost children, such as Andrew, to these diseases. In recent years researchers around the world have used patients' tumor tissue to generate dozens of cell lines and mouse models to study the basic biology of pediatric brain cancers. The time is ripe. In the dawn of precision medicine, which aims to customize disease treatment to the individual patient, genetics and basic science findings suggest why past trials may have failed and are guiding future and ongoing efforts to identify effective therapeutics for these devastating diseases.

Michelle Monje, an assistant professor of neurology at Stanford University, first encountered DIPG around 2002 as an MD/PhD student there. Working with her clinical mentor to care for a nine-year-old girl dying of DIPG, it was "the first time I'd come upon a disease we had no idea how to treat," Monje says. "I felt so close to this patient and was devastated by my inability to help her."

Back then there was little molecular data on DIPG. No animal models. No cell cultures. Generating such research tools requires tumor samples from patients. Yet since MRI scans can reliably diagnose typical DIPG and getting brain stem tissue is not trivial, biopsies were rarely done. With precious little tumor tissue to study in the lab, Monje says, research progress on DIPG had stalled for decades.

The tide started turning by 2007, when a team of surgeons in France reported safely obtaining biopsy samples from 24 children with DIPG using stereotactic techniques that use computer imaging to guide needle placement. That study invigorated longstanding efforts by a pediatric neuro-oncologist Mark Kieran, clinical director of the Brain Tumor Center at Dana-Farber/Boston Children's Cancer and Blood Disorders Center, who had spent years pushing for DIPG biopsies in the U.S., initially without success.

By that time technological advances had made it possible to read DNA sequences from tiny bits of tissue, giving further impetus for a tricky surgical procedure now shown to be safe in trained hands. The Boston team began offering patients genomic sequencing of their tumors biopsied at diagnosis and relapse, to "see how the tumor is evolving and redirect the appropriate drugs to it," Kieran says. Tumor profiles could help determine which patients might benefit from a newer class of drugs called targeted therapies, which hit specific proteins in the tumor rather than just kill off any dividing cell. Targeted therapies are a cornerstone of precision medicine.

Since 2009 researchers at Dana–Farber have sequenced brain tumors in nearly 1,000 children. Among kids with tumors classified as a low-grade glioma, up to 10 percent have a mutation in a gene called *BRAF* that is seen in some adult skin tumors. A few years ago, 32 children from Europe and North America with *BRAF*-positive gliomas entered a clinical trial of dabrafenib, a targeted therapy approved for melanoma patients with this mutation. At a conference in Copenhagen earlier this month, Kieran reported that 23 of the 32 kids improved on the BRAF-inhibiting drug—a response rate high enough that his team is offering continued therapy to trial participants with the mutation.

In 2012 Kieran and collaborators launched a clinical trial to biopsy tumors of children with DIPG, test them for several molecular markers and, based on the results, assign one of four treatment strategies. Two years ago a team led by Sabine Mueller, a pediatric neuro-oncologist at the University of California, San Francisco, initiated another DIPG trial. This study probes patient tumors using a more sophisticated technique, whole exome sequencing, which scours the entire protein-encoding portion of the genome rather than just checking for pre-specified markers. Based on each patient's tumor profile, the U.C. San Francisco team proposed up to four drugs that seem appropriate. It will take another one to two years to see if the drugs help.

Although helpful for some individuals, precision medicine is expensive, and some scientists suspect it may only modestly improve the lives of cancer patients in general. Cells within a single tumor can acquire different mutations, such that "even if there is an effective agent, it is likely to have limited benefit because molecular pathways that are active in other parts of the tumor will lead to tumor growth from different clones of tumor cells," researchers wrote in a *New England Journal of Medicine* commentary published in September. And without specific drugs approved for DIPG, there is ongoing debate about whether biopsies offer real benefit to these patients.

Some labs have taken a less controversial route to DIPG samples–obtaining them as legacy gifts from families who agree to donate tumor tissue once their child passes. Smith, the Michigan mom, learned about legacy gifts through an online DIPG support group in spring of 2008, a half year after her son Andrew was diagnosed. Reading that post about removing the brain after death and donating the tissue "was horrifying to me," Smith recalls. "But I understood [that without patient samples] there was no way for researchers to look at this tumor." She shared the idea on a Yahoo group for DIPG families that she and her friend moderate. In November 2008, a mother from the Yahoo list called Smith in a panic. Her daughter was in her final hours, and the family wanted her tumor tissue donated but hadn't made arrangements.

Autopsy tissue donations are logistically challenging. Once a child passes, the brain needs to be removed, with tumor tissue placed into sterile tubes, within six hours. Yet patients tend to die at home, far from the medical center, sometimes in the middle of the night or during a snowstorm on a holiday weekend. Some labs book on-call service from a tissue recovery team close to where the child lives. To have the biggest impact, samples should go to labs that can receive and process them the same day.

As Smith helped other families arrange tumor donations, she got to know some of the leading DIPG researchers, including Monje, who had just worked out a way to culture cells from autopsy tissue and use those cells to create mouse models of DIPG. In July 2011 Smith learned of a seven-year-old girl named McKenna, who was battling DIPG. Smith and Monje worked with the family and "made sure we had the required documents when the time came," says McKenna's mother, Kristine Wetzel, a high school teacher in Huntington Beach, Calif.

McKenna faded suddenly, and the family decided to donate her tumor tissue within an hour of her death. Although painful, the decision was "surprisingly comforting," Wetzel says. "It was a way to fight back against the monster that had stolen our daughter." The Wetzels have since helped other DIPG families with tumor donations and created a foundation to raise awareness and fund research in pediatric brain cancer. The foundation covers the cost of tissue donations to Monje's lab and pays for a technician who maintains the lab's DIPG cultures and has shipped samples to some 80 labs around the world. Support varies but usually amounts to about $100,000 per year, Monje says.

Autopsy tissue donations have "transformed the research landscape from an unapproachable problem, due to lack of material for research, to an unprecedented analysis of the DIPG genome," says neurobiologist Suzanne Baker, who helps lead the Neurobiology and Brain Tumor Program at St. Jude Children's Research Hospital.

A wave of papers by Baker, Kiernan and others at Washington University School of Medicine in St. Louis and elsewhere revealed a surprise. Although DIPG has a gene signature distinct from other brain cancers, the rare childhood tumors share one striking feature: Nearly 80 percent of them have mutations in a gene that codes for a protein called histone H3. Histone proteins are like spools around which DNA wraps. A key player in epigenetics–the study of biological mechanisms that turn genes on or off–histones influence how easily DNA is accessed by enzymes that translate genetic code into working proteins. "Histone H3 is so fundamental...I would think lots of cancers would have these mutations," Baker says. Yet they seem to be unique to DIPG and about a third of non–brain stem tumors in kids.

The genetic insights could not have come at a better time. Whereas some labs were busy plumbing whole genome sequencing data from DIPG tumor cells, others were testing potential drugs in cell cultures and mouse models generated from patient brain tumor samples. The idea was to carefully vet compounds in the lab before choosing which ones to test in a longer, costlier clinical trial. The approach is not revolutionary. Generally it is "the way you do medical research," Monje says. But for DIPG, "we'd been unable to do this" for decades because there had been no cell cultures or experimental mice modeling the disease.

The situation improved in 2010 when Charles Keller, then at Oregon Health & Science University, organized a global screening effort. By then many labs were creating cell cultures from DIPG tumor tissue. As co-chair of a committee proposing drugs for DIPG clinical trials, Keller rallied the Monje lab and 12 other groups to pool resources for a collaborative study. His group dispensed 83 potential drugs onto well plates and sent them to the other labs for testing. At these far-flung labs researchers loaded the plates with DIPG cell cultures and looked for wells that turned blue–a chemical indication that the drug was killing tumor cells. Top drug candidates also improved survival in mice with implanted DIPG tumors.

In addition, the labs purified genetic material from their DIPG cell lines and sent DNA and RNA samples to Oregon for sequencing to establish a clear tie between the cells' gene glitch and drug response. Checking for these connections is key, Keller says, because many drugs that looked promising based on mutations in the DIPG cells showed no effect in the cellular assays.

But there emerged a winner–a drug called panobinostat, which inhibits enzymes that chemically modify histone proteins. Coincidentally, the U.S. Food and Drug Administration approved panobinostat as a treatment for another cancer, multiple myeloma, as the global screening manuscript went to press in *Nature Medicine.* The results helped launch a clinical trial of panobinostat that opened for enrollment in May. Led by Monje, this trial will measure side effects and determine the best doses of the drug for treating children with DIPG. Panobinostat is not going to be a silver bullet, however. The lab data showed some DIPG cells develop resistance to the drug, suggesting it will need to be combined with other therapies to achieve a survival benefit in patients, Monje says.

One challenge with panobinostat is shared by many brain cancer therapies—delivering them effectively into the brain. "Many drugs don't cross the blood–brain barrier so they are not getting to the tumor," says U.C. San Francisco's Mueller. Some researchers are using a procedure called convection-enhanced delivery to place drugs through small catheters directly into the brain tumor. Others are using nanotechnology to reformulate drugs so they can be more specific and durable—for example, by inserting molecular tags that direct the drug to molecules found uniquely on the tumor. It is possible that good drugs for DIPG already exist, Mueller says, but "we just don't know how to deliver them correctly." She is planning a future trial using convection-enhanced delivery of panobinostat in kids with DIPG.

In the meantime Monje's lab and other groups are doing additional drug screens with epigenetic agents and combination regimens, and Keller founded a nonprofit cancer biotech to speed the movement of candidate drugs from basic science research to clinical testing. Each year his team organizes a weeklong crash course to teach families about pediatric brain cancers and explain how tumor tissue donations are driving research.

Some families make regular visits to the lab to see their child's cells under the microscope. Wetzel's family visited Monje's lab eight to nine months after their daughter died of DIPG. "The first time I saw McKenna's cells, I started crying uncontrollably," Wetzel says. "I wanted to take every petri dish...and throw it against the wall, to the destroy the cell line like it had destroyed my daughter."

Now, after trips to the lab about once a year, Wetzel feels differently. "I see it as McKenna's last stand...her gift to the world and to children who will follow her. If McKenna can't be here, let her make the world a better place in the one way she now can. It helps us to think there was some purpose to her death."

About the Author

Esther Landhuis is a freelance science and health journalist based in the San Francisco Bay Area. Follow her on Twitter @elandhuis.

A Shot against Cancer

By Karen Weintraub

Michelle Boyer got an extra six years of life. Karen Koehler had six nearly symptom-free years, thinking she had beaten her diagnosis. And Doug Olson has officially been declared "cured" more than a decade after he thought he was out of options. These people are three of thousands who, in the past 10 years, have experienced both the promise and the challenges of an approach to treating cancer by manipulating the immune system. Instead of attacking cancer from the outside—slicing out tumors or dousing the body with toxic chemicals or radiation—immunotherapy energizes the complex and highly interactive cells and molecular signals of its defense networks to do the job from the inside.

Like those older approaches, immunotherapy has become one of the pillars of cancer care for blood cancers such as Olson's and Koehler's and for melanoma like Boyer had, as well as for bladder, breast and lung cancer—the last being America's biggest cancer killer, responsible for more than 130,000 deaths in 2021.

The transformation has been dramatic, from just reaching oncologists' radar a decade ago to beginning to catch on five to six years ago. "There has been a 180-degree change in the center of gravity in both cancer research and clinical oncology practice," says Ira Mellman, vice president of cancer immunology at Genentech in California. Immunotherapy "has become the standard of care in lung cancer, which not long ago was treated with either surgery or chemotherapy, or both." The results so far have been encouraging but far from universal, and progress has not been as fast as "a lot of us anticipated or hoped," says Stanley Riddell, who researches immunotherapies at the Fred Hutchinson Cancer Research Center in Seattle. "Curing cancer's not easy." Given now to tens of thousands of patients, the treatments provide near miracles in some cases, dashed hopes in others.

Doctors are still at the beginning of understanding which patients will be helped by immunotherapy and which will not. Factors at play seem to include how many T cells have already made it into the tumor microenvironment, how hard it is for the immune system to recognize cancer cells, and even the patient's makeup of gut microbes, Riddell says. Former President Jimmy Carter was almost 91 in August 2015 when he announced that his melanoma, the most lethal form of skin cancer, had spread to his liver and brain. News outlets readied their obituaries. But Carter received radiation and then an immunotherapy drug that releases the brakes cancer can put on the immune system, called checkpoint inhibitors. By December of that year, all evidence of his tumors was gone, and he has since celebrated his 97th birthday. It is likely that he saw such incredible benefits because his cancer resulted from years in the sun, which triggered a wide variety of mutations. That and damage from radiation made his cancer cells easier for his immune system to recognize once immunotherapy lifted the brakes.

Boyer, a Seattle resident, was diagnosed with advanced melanoma in her 20s, so her cancer was probably the product of fewer mutations. In 2013 she started a series of revolutionary treatments–some of which first became available in 2011–that prompted her immune system to identify, attack and shrink the tumors. But even unleashing the immune system was not enough to elicit a full-blown attack, and she died in 2019 at age 32.

Beyond the mutational burden of an individual's cancer, doctors do not know much about who will or will not do well on these drugs. They have looked for years for molecular markers that could be predictive, but they have not had much success. While the hunt continues, researchers are testing drug combinations and other approaches, such as vaccinations, to stretch the benefits to more patients. Such combinations are needed both because cancers are complicated, being the product of various genetic mutations, and because, as immunologists have learned, the immune system has multiple layers of defense and offense. "You need really to combine, to synergize different modes of action," says Özlem Türeci, a cancer immunotherapy pioneer who co-founded BioNTech, now known for collaborating with Pfizer on a COVID vaccine. "Different task forces with nonredundant, partially overlapping modes of action are combined. This is how the immune system has naturally evolved."

Liquid Success

The dream of fighting cancer with the immune system dates back at least 125 years to William Coley of New York City, a physician who injected some of his cancer patients with bacteria in an effort to jump-start their body's natural healing powers. Coley's approach was taken up by a few other doctors. But it gradually fell out of favor after his death in 1936, to be replaced by advances in chemotherapy and, later, hormone and antibody treatments, which showed more consistent results in a greater number of patients.

The idea of boosting the immune system never entirely lost its appeal, though, in part because it was promoted by the Cancer Research Institute, a New York City–based philanthropy started in 1953 by Coley's daughter. The field was not well respected for decades, Türeci says, but in more recent years, as HIV research has led to a deeper understanding of the immune system and genetics has enabled a more in-depth view of tumors, cancer investigators have stocked their arsenal with potent immunological weapons.

Among the most attractive targets for those weapons have been cancers of the circulatory and lymphatic systems such as leukemia and lymphoma. These diseases occur when various kinds of progenitor cells, called stem cells, that normally give rise to red and white blood cells (among other tissues) develop mutations and grow uncontrollably, crowding out healthy cells and robbing the body of their vital functions. Many of these so-called liquid tumors form when something goes wrong with a part of the immune system called B cells. Normally B cells generate antibodies against bacteria and viruses. (B cells also help to coordinate various other immune responses, along with another group of cells, T cells.) But when B cells become cancerous, they destroy the body from the inside out.

In the late 20th century investigators developed the biological equivalent of a guided missile that attached itself to a B cell protein (CD20) found on the cells' surface at a specific, late stage of their existence. Dubbed rituximab, this monoclonal antibody signaled T cells to do something they do not usually do: attack and destroy these older, CD20-bearing B cells. CD20 is not a cancer-specific marker, though, and it appears on normal B cells as well as dangerous ones, so the drug killed both healthy and cancerous B cells. It turns out, however, that most people can live without B cells. (The same is not true of T cells, as the death of millions of people infected with T cell–targeting HIV tragically demonstrates.) And after the drug wore off, most patients eventually started making B cells on their own again from the stockpile of stem cells in their bone marrow. Clinical trials in the 1990s demonstrated that the combination of chemotherapy and rituximab was particularly effective against B cell–based cancers.

For Koehler, a retired special education teacher from Park Ridge, N.J., leukemia originated with mutant B cells, but rituximab made her very sick and seemed only partially effective, so she stopped taking it. In addition, tests indicated her cancer would resist standard chemotherapy. Because her malignancy was rapidly getting worse, her doctors suggested a then-experimental immune treatment custom-designed to fight her form of leukemia. She agreed. The goal was to destroy all of Koehler's B cells, as rituximab would, but with two key differences. A different protein on the B cells, CD19, was the mark. And rather than using a drug to paint a target on that protein, attracting killer T cells already in Koehler's body, doctors took a more direct approach. They removed some of her T cells and genetically engineered them to attack CD19 without any prompting.

Investigators call these turbocharged cells chimeric antigen receptor T cells, or CAR Ts. They display some of the characteristics of both T cells and B cells in much the same way that ancient mythological creatures called chimeras were supposed to be made up of different animals. The U.S. Food and Drug Administration has approved a handful of CAR Ts so far, directed at CD19 or other cell surface markers. Previously CAR Ts had been used mostly as last-ditch therapies after others failed, but now they are being pushed earlier in the disease course, when patients–and their immune systems–are likely to be healthier and more responsive. Riddell says he is optimistic that improvements will come from treating patients earlier and perhaps from using combinations of CAR Ts designed to target both CD19 and CD20, as well as other antigens. He notes that among three recent trials in people with relapsed lymphoma, patients fared better if they received CAR Ts than the current standard-of-care bone marrow transplant.

Olson also volunteered for a CAR T trial long before the treatment was approved. One of the first three patients to sign up at the University of Pennsylvania for the experimental therapy in 2010, he saw it as his last chance to beat the chronic lymphocytic leukemia he had already lived with for 14 years. A few weeks after his infusion, he ended up in the hospital with flulike symptoms, one of three major side effects of the therapy. So many cancer cells were dying off so quickly that their removal was damaging his kidneys. After three days he stabilized, and his oncologist David Porter brought him some good news: already 19 percent of the T cells in his bone marrow consisted of the CD19-targeting CAR T cells. A month after the infusion they made up 100 percent of his T cells, and there was no sign of cancer left at all.

Olson says he has had no more side effects from the therapy, although his CAR T cells kept killing off his healthy B cells, so he needs monthly infusions of IVIG, antibodies that help fight off disease. In a study published in February 2022 in the journal *Nature Medicine*, researchers at Penn showed that some of his T cells and those of another patient treated around the same time, who has since died of COVID, still bore the CAR T signatures nearly a decade later and were able to kill leukemia cells in a lab dish. The CAR T cells that remained in Olson's body had transformed from killer T cells into the more sentrylike $CD4^+$ T cells. This suggests that patients like Olson have two distinct phases of response to CAR Ts: one in which killer T cells attack tumor cells and a second in which these $CD4^+$ T cells maintain long-term remission by patrolling for any lingering cancer.

That evolution might not happen in everyone. Perhaps that is why Koehler's remission did not lead to her being cured. By 2016, more than a year after a single infusion of CAR Ts derived from her own, altered cells, Koehler, then 59, was convinced she had hit the immunotherapy jackpot. Within a month of her treatment, scans showed no signs of cancer in her body. But she had already suffered through another of the potentially serious side effects of CAR Ts. The night she received her reengineered cells, a so-called cytokine storm landed her in intensive care. This reaction occurs when many more T cells than usual are activated at once, triggering a flood of chemical signals, called cytokines, that the immune system uses to communicate. The result can be a life-threatening frenzy of activity in which immune cells destroy healthy tissues, causing multiorgan failure. Riddell compares it to an explosion of inflammation inside the body. Koehler remained in intensive care for eight days, half of which she was in a coma and totally unresponsive. She has no memory of that time, but at one point, Koehler, an avid golfer, was so delusional that she asked nurses for help packing lunch for a pair of famous golfers.

By the time she got out of the hospital, in early March 2015, Koehler was incredibly weak but rebounding fast. A bone marrow test showed no evidence of cancer, and three weeks later she was back on the golf course. Koehler was one of the first clinical trial volunteers to endure this kind of dramatic, life-threatening cytokine storm. She says she was also the last of her doctor's patients to end up in intensive care. Today when Koehler, a volunteer, counsels patients about to get CAR T therapy, she tells them they will stay in an apartment across the street from the hospital and might have to be admitted for a few days. But "no one really gets sick," she says. "No one thinks they're in Wyoming," like she did during her delusions.

Another challenge with CAR T is its incredible price tag. The therapy routinely costs $375,000 to $475,000. Penn's Carl June, in announcing the February 2022 *Nature Medicine* study Olson was part of, said the cost is high but less expensive than trying to keep someone alive on other, less effective therapies.

Efforts are also underway to bring costs down. Until now, CAR Ts have been given mainly at academic medical centers after being manufactured in small research labs. But 140 biotechnology companies and every major pharmaceutical company, impressed by the therapy's success, have gotten in on the act and should soon be producing the cells at larger scale for lower cost, based on improved manufacturing technologies and market competition, says Michel Sadelain, director of the center for cell engineering at Memorial Sloan Kettering Cancer Center in New York City.

Olson's results suggest that few cell clones–just three make up the majority in his case–are long-lasting. If researchers can figure out what is special about those rare cells and just deliver those, instead of millions of others, the cost of therapy will drop substantially, Sadelain says. Researchers are also trying to develop cell therapy approaches that would be less personalized and more off the shelf but still effective, which could cost far less.

The other major challenge facing CAR T treatment is translating its success from liquid cancers to solid tumors–the kind that form lumps in breast, prostate, lung, skin and other tissues. CAR Ts may have a hard time leaving the bloodstream to find a solid tumor, Mellman explains. In the blood, the liquid tumor cells are relatively easy for the CAR Ts to locate. Even more important, CAR Ts for liquid cancers can be targeted specifically and safely to the affected cell lineages. There are no comparable cell lineages in solid tumors; they do not express surface molecules that are not also expressed by normal tissues. But Mellman sees tremendous long-term potential for this type of immune system manipulation. "What we're looking at now with CAR Ts are still preliminary, almost crude approaches as compared to what I think will be possible when you can bring the full power of cell engineering to bear on the problem," he says.

Solid State

Solid tumors pose other difficulties for immune treatments. They are often surrounded by a matrix of connective and other tissues, which blocks cells from entering the malignant mass. In addition, the internal pressure of a solid tumor is typically higher than that of its surroundings, which tends to flush out the chemical signals that the immune system uses to flag aberrant cells—not to mention many drugs.

Yet these tumors have shown some vulnerability. In 2011 the FDA approved a monoclonal antibody called ipilimumab to treat advanced cases of melanoma. Unlike traditional therapy, ipilimumab is not designed to kill tumors directly; rather it releases the biological brakes that some cancers are able to put on the immune system, freeing the body's defenses to do a better job. (Carter was treated with a second-generation checkpoint inhibitor called pembrolizumab.)

Melanoma has a nasty habit of defrauding immune system cells. The clumps of cancer cells have an assortment of malformed proteins on their surface, which T cells are supposed to spot, swarm around and destroy before the aberrant growth has a chance to get any bigger. But every now and then a nascent tumor develops a way to send out chemical signals that tell the T cells all is well and to stand down.

In effect, the cancer cells have hijacked a normal feature of the immune system: a safety mechanism that tamps down the body's rampaging defense cells before they start damaging healthy tissue. More specifically, this safety mechanism consists of a series of checkpoints, or gateways, that either rally defense cells to attack or turn them off, depending on which chemical signals are present. (If the checkpoints ever got stuck in the "open" position, the ensuing immune reaction would probably kill a person faster than any malignant growth could.)

Cancer cells have workarounds that enable them to hide from the immune system by disabling T cells that could kill them. Blocking that false signal with ipilimumab or other checkpoint inhibitors reawakens the immune cells, allowing them once again to zero in on their targets. Ipilimumab soon proved effective in lung cancer as well as melanoma, and pharmaceutical companies began developing other drugs that used the same strategy.

A 2015 study in the *New England Journal of Medicine* showed that more melanoma patients did better when given two checkpoint inhibitors instead of one. Still, doctors are not good at predicting who will respond to which checkpoint inhibitor or combination of treatments, so some patients have to keep experimenting with different therapies. Today about half the people treated with combination checkpoint inhibitors are alive for at least six years after their treatment. To confuse matters even more, some tumors that appear to attract few T cells still respond to checkpoint inhibitors, whereas the drugs sometimes have no effect on other tumors that contain lots of T cells–suggesting the cancer is playing other tricks.

That has made picking an effective solid tumor treatment for a particular individual a matter of trial and error, as Boyer's experience shows. Two years after she had surgery to remove the cancerous mole from her back, Boyer learned that the melanoma had returned and was spreading throughout her lungs and chest. Because the growths were too large to be cut out, Boyer agreed, on the advice of her physicians, to take part in a clinical trial at the beginning of 2013 in which she would be injected with high doses of interleukin-2 (IL-2), one of dozens of different chemical signals that help to boost the immune system's ability to fight cancer. At first the drug seemed to stop the growth of Boyer's tumors, but after three months scans showed that the cancer was on the move again.

Boyer opted for a second clinical trial, this time pairing the recently approved checkpoint inhibitor ipilimumab with still another immune-signaling molecule known as IL-21. Within a few weeks, however, the side effects of the IL-21 treatment (nausea, diarrhea and unbearable pain) had become so disabling that Boyer had to stop getting the injections, although she continued receiving the ipilimumab. By the end of 2013 some of the cancerous spots had started to expand, so her medical team opted for radiation to try to limit the growth. By spring of the following year a few of these tumors were smaller, but new ones had appeared on her head and in her breast.

Surgery dispatched the lump in her breast, and two other immune-boosting therapies seemed to hold the rest of her tumors in check for a while. By January 2015, however, it had become clear that she needed another plan of action–new spots had begun to grow in her brain, breast and abdomen. A month later she entered a clinical trial that combined yet another checkpoint inhibitor with a drug that is supposed to slow tumor growth. Boyer's cancerous spots remained stable for a while but eventually worsened.

The treatments battered Boyer's body. By late 2016 she was spending her nights and many of her days in a plush loveseat to rest her back. During her sixth round of treatment, she was able to work most mornings in her job as a structural engineer. Otherwise she entertained herself by playing video games–*Call of Duty* was her favorite. She did not regret the game of Whac-A-Mole her doctors were playing with her cancer. "It seems to me that some of these treatments maybe slowed down the growth a little bit," she said in 2016. One of her doctors, Boyer remembered, "said part of the game for melanoma was not necessarily finding the right treatment now but keeping yourself alive long enough until they find the right treatment."

Unfortunately for Boyer, they didn't. Her June 13, 2019, obituary notes that she had participated in clinical trials, "hoping to find treatments for future patients." She was incredibly grateful for the outstanding medical care she had received at the Seattle Cancer Care Alliance and the University of Washington Medical Center, and she "wanted people to know that she was at peace with her death."

Looking Ahead

Immunotherapy probably bought Boyer extra time. That is promising for cancer researchers, even if the ending was not fit for a fairy tale. Investigators no longer need to worry about whether their research will eventually help someone; now they can spend their time making effective treatments better. "We need to find the boundaries and limitations" and figure out how to work with the immune system to be more effective against a wider range of cancer types, Mellman says, but "this is an incredibly inspiring and thrilling way to do science."

Eventually the process of selecting an immune treatment will become more logical, based on the characteristic immunological profile of a patient's tumor, Mellman believes. A patient with a solid tumor will first have it biopsied to look for the presence of T cells. If enough T cells are in the tumor, the person will likely be given a single checkpoint inhibitor or maybe several inhibitors. (At present, the FDA has approved eight checkpoint inhibitors, with more under development.) If the tumor has not already attracted many T cells or if the T cells are unable to enter the tumor, scientists will have to find other approaches to generate, attract or facilitate the entry of tumor-specific T cells.

Researchers are also considering how to use standard cancer care, including radiation, targeted agents (such as mutant K-Ras inhibitors) and chemotherapy, to boost the immune response. Killing a number of tumor cells with lower doses of chemotherapy or radiation should release lots of cellular debris from the tumor, thereby alerting the immune system to send T cells to whatever abnormal growth remains. (Getting the balance right may be tricky because too much chemotherapy and radiation have also been shown to suppress parts of the immune system.) Then the addition of a checkpoint inhibitor might be able to effectively fight the weakened cancer before it has a chance to recover.

Other combinatory approaches may soon include cancer vaccines. Türeci's BioNTech, among other companies, has been working on experimental vaccines that one day will be able to spur the immune system to attack cancer. So far BioNTech has made the best advances in treating colon cancer patients who have had surgery but are at high risk of recurrence and with personalized vaccines designed to attack an individual's melanoma. Vaccines can trigger the body to generate a larger army of T cells, Türeci says, and then checkpoint inhibitors empower these T cells to roam freely in the body and attack lingering tumor cells.

Adding a vaccine might also help patients who got some response, like Boyer, but not a long-term benefit from a checkpoint inhibitor, Türeci says. Messenger RNA, the same vehicle used in BioNTech's potent COVID vaccine, is a natural tool for immunotherapy, she adds. It amplifies the effect of the antigen by triggering a stronger immune response than earlier generations of cancer vaccines , which proved too weak. It is also viable for a personalized vaccine because one mRNA can easily be exchanged for another. "There is a new era for vaccines now," she says.

Other researchers are manipulating T cell receptors, or TCRs, to encourage them to attack cancer cells, or using tumor-infiltrating lymphocytes, or TILs, which are taken out of the body, amplified in number in a lab and then reinfused. Steven Rosenberg of the National Institutes of Health has shown that about 15 to 20 percent of patients get a dramatic response from TILs, living as long as 15 years after treatment so far. "The question is, How do we make that a bigger pot?" Riddell asks.

Researchers are learning more about T cell exhaustion, a state in which the immune soldiers seem to just give up the fight. Single-cell sequencing is allowing insights at a more granular level than ever before. And gene editing is enabling scientists to put that new knowledge to good use, Riddell says. So new advances are bound to come. As he notes, it took 50 years to optimize chemotherapy, and checkpoint blockades and CAR Ts have been around for only a decade. "The potency of the immune system for eradicating cancers is really quite remarkable," Riddell says. If cancer is a mountain range, "we've climbed the first peak, but there are more peaks."

All these new therapies and combinations will be expensive, of course. The global market for oncology drugs is expected to top $250 billion a year by 2025, according to IQVIA, a health-care data company. Insurers and the public will not be willing or able to indefinitely combine drugs that can run to hundreds of thousands of dollars or more per patient. So companies are looking at manufacturing improvements, lower doses and shorter treatment times, among other approaches, to reduce treatment costs. But it is hard to argue with the value that more cures could provide.

Koehler, now 65, got six great years from her engineered T cells. Other than the IVIG infusions and regular checkups, she was able to lead a normal life. "I felt phenomenal," she says. And it lasted so long that she "got a little cocky," thinking her cancer days were over. But scans in late 2021 showed her leukemia had come roaring back. As of this writing, she was still waiting for her doctor to finish analyzing her blood work and recommend next steps.

"If we could do the CAR T again, I'd drive to the hospital right now," she says. Doctors still have her cells, but CAR T is not yet approved for second-time use, and it is not clear whether her current cancer cells have the same CD19 receptors on their surface. Instead Koehler might end up on a drug called ibrutinib, an immunotherapy that is often given to treat chronic lymphocytic leukemia–but she would have to take it for the rest of her life. She told her doctor she would rather have another round of CAR T therapy: "I don't want maintenance. I want you to knock it out again." Cancer doctors hope immunotherapy will soon allow them to give many more patients extra years of high-quality life.

About the Author

Karen Weintraub is a staff writer at USA Today, *where she covers COVID, vaccine development and other health issues.*

Are We Innately Immune to Cancer?

By Mark Lowdell

The study of cancer immunity has been a global challenge since William Coley first treated patients with his eponymous toxin in the late 19th century. As our understanding of the immune system has evolved, its role in the fight against cancer has become increasingly apparent. There have been some monumental milestones that helped shape cancer treatment as it stands today, including Steven Rosenberg's trials of tumor-infiltrating lymphocytes in the 1980s, Hans Kolb's cure of leukemia with donor T cells in the 1990s, and the discovery of checkpoint blockade, which led to Jim Allison's 2018 Nobel Prize and the explosion of the field of immunotherapy.

The focus on immunotherapy puts us at risk for forgetting that the principal role of the immune system is tumor surveillance: the elimination of developing diseases before we are even aware of the danger. Cancer arises from the uncontrolled growth of tumor cells, which have evaded immune surveillance, and immunotherapies are aimed at restoring the body's natural anticancer responses. Nevertheless, despite some groundbreaking results, current immunotherapies remain effective in only a minority of patients.

The reason is that most such therapies target only one of the two sides of the immune system, the adaptive response, and not the innate response. Now many immunotherapists are beginning to understand that broadening our therapeutic options to target the innate response as well will give patients the best chance of beating their disease.

Adaptive immunity, also referred to as acquired immunity, is an antigen-specific immune response that can kill cancer cells and then generate an immunological memory of each tumor-related antigen. This creates a reservoir of immune cells that are able to respond to cancer cells expressing the same specific antigen should it reappear. Adaptive immunity consists of T and B lymphocytes, which lyse tumor cells and generate antibodies to some of the tumor antigens. The process of adaptive immunity is the foundation of vaccinations such as the HPV vaccine, which targets the virus responsible for most cases of cervical cancer.

Why is innate immunotherapy likely to improve outcomes? Innate immunity is our body's first line of defense against infection and cancer. Around 10 percent of the lymphocytes in our peripheral bloodstream are part of the innate response, and 95 percent of those are natural killer (NK) cells. Each of these innate killer cells can recognize, target and kill harmful cells through recognition of proteins and glycoproteins, which are expressed on "stressed" cells, such as tumor and virally infected cells.

In contrast to the adaptive immunity's antigen-specific T cell responses, the innate system is relatively nonspecific and can provide a rapid response. Whereas some of the earliest cellular immunotherapy trials in cancer were directed at innate immunity, many believed that the innate response is inadequate for the control of cancer and instead redirected therapies to focus on the T cell–mediated adaptive immunity.

Clinically, innate and adaptive immunity work together to protect us from infection and cancer, yet our understanding of innate immunity remains relatively poor compared with the adaptive responses. This is partly because adaptive immunity was not discovered until the 1970s and partly because of the technical difficulties in studying NK cell biology compared with T and B cells. The importance of the innate response is accepted in invertebrates, which lack adaptive immunity. It is clearly essential for humans, too.

Human NK cells are evolutionarily conserved and even share many molecules with NK cells from invertebrates such as leeches and sea urchins. From the early days of HIV infection, we saw that patients with a fundamentally damaged adaptive immune system were still protected by their innate immune system and succumbed only to some intracellular bacterial infections and rare tumors. They did not die from common infections or uncontrolled tumors.

Today we have a great deal of supporting evidence for the importance of NK cells and the innate response in protection from cancer. Cancer cells are constantly arising in our bodies as a consequence of random genetic mutations, some of which give a cell a survival or proliferation advantage. These random changes are mostly novel and have never been presented to the adaptive immune system. The only cells able to detect the "stress" signals of a tumor cell that is dividing too frequently are NK cells, which can eliminate tumor cells before they become a clinically detectable cancer.

A Japanese study published in 2000 measured the resting NK cell response to a single cancer cell line in more than 3,500 healthy people on a single day of their life and then followed them all for more than 11 years. Those with the weakest resting NK cell function on the single test day had a statistically significantly increased incidence of succumbing to any form of cancer over the period of follow-up. The importance of innate immune surveillance is also seen in NK cell–deficient mice, which generate malignant lymphomas spontaneously.

Far from being the poor, unsophisticated relative of the adaptive immune response, innate immunity is central to survival. As we increase our understanding of the innate immune response and discover how to best manipulate it, NK cell therapies alone will provide even greater advances in immunotherapy for cancer. Alongside treatments involving the adaptive immune response, they will enable us to target cancer better than ever before."

The views expressed are those of the author(s) and are not necessarily those of Scientific American.

About the Author

Mark Lowdell is chief scientific officer of INmune Bio, an immunotherapy company developing treatments to reprogram the innate immune system to fight disease.

Darwin's Ideas on Evolution Drive a Radical New Approach to Cancer Drug Use

By James DeGregori, Robert Gatenby

This year at least 31,000 men in the U.S. will be diagnosed with prostate cancer that has spread to other parts of their body, such as bones and lymph nodes. Most of them will be treated by highly skilled and experienced oncologists, who have access to 52 drugs approved to treat this condition. Yet eventually more than three quarters of these men will succumb to their illness.

Cancers that have spread, known as metastatic disease, are rarely curable. The reasons that patients die despite effective treatment are many, but they all trace back to an idea popularized in 1859 by Charles Darwin to explain the rise and fall of species of birds and tortoises. Today we call it evolution.

Think of a cancer cell like Darwin's Galápagos finches, which had slightly different beaks on various islands. Finches eat seeds, and seeds on each island had different shapes or other characteristics. The bird with a beak shape best matched to the local seed got the most food and had the most offspring, which also had that particular beak shape. Birds with less adaptive beaks did not make it. This natural selection ensured that different finch species, with various beaks, evolved on each island. The key is that when two groups of critters compete in the same small space, the one better adapted to the environment wins out.

Cancer cells evolve in a similar manner. In normal tissue, regular noncancer cells thrive because they are a good fit for the biochemical growth signals, nutrients and physical cues they get from surrounding healthy tissue. If a mutation creates a cancer cell poorly adapted for those surroundings, it does not stand much chance initially: normal cells outcompete it for resources. But if the surroundings are further damaged by inflammation—

sometimes a growing cancer can cause this itself—or old age, the cancer cell does better and starts to outcompete normal cells that used to crowd it out. The change in the surroundings ultimately determines a cancer cell's success.

This is a theory we call adaptive oncogenesis, and we have found evidence that supports it in the way cancer takes off when we change its cellular environment in experimental animals, although the internal workings of the cancer cell have not changed. Doctors have also observed this acceleration of cancer in humans with tissue-disturbing ailments such as inflammatory bowel disease. The overall implication is that we can best understand cancer by looking at its surroundings rather than solely focusing on the mutations inside a cell. By reducing tissue alterations caused by processes such as inflammation, we can restore a more normal environment and—as we have shown in animal studies—prevent cancer from gaining a competitive edge.

Our evolutionary perspective also has inspired a different approach to cancer therapy, one that we have successfully tested in small clinical trials. Doctors dump a lot of chemotherapy drugs on a cancer in an effort to kill every last trace of the threat, and at first this often looks like it works. The tumor shrinks or goes away. But then it comes back and is resistant to the drugs that once killed these cells, akin to crop-destroying insects that evolve resistance to pesticides. In a clinical trial with prostate cancer patients, one of us (Gatenby) tried an alternative to the scorched-earth approach, applying only enough chemo to keep the tumor tiny without killing it entirely. The goal was to maintain a small population of vulnerable chemosensitive cells. That population did well enough to prevent cells with an unwanted new trait—chemoresistance—from taking over. In a group of patients in which tumors usually start growing uncontrollably after 13 months, this regimen has kept tumors under control for 34 months on average—with less than half the standard drug dose.

The results of our prevention and therapeutic strategies may point to a way to ward off cancer before it becomes a danger to life and limb and to save many patients for whom a regimen of giant, toxic drug doses has failed.

Why Do We Get Cancer?

If you asked almost any doctor or cancer researcher, "Why is aging, smoking or radiation exposure associated with cancer?" you would probably get a short answer: "These things cause mutations." This assessment is partly true. Exposure to cigarette smoke or radiation does cause mutations in our DNA, and mutations do accumulate in our cells throughout life. The mutations can provide cells with new properties, such as hyperactive growth signals for cell divisions, reduced death rates or even an increased ability to invade surrounding tissue.

Yet this simple explanation, focused on changes within cells, overlooks the fact that a major driver of evolutionary change in any single cell—or in entire collections of them, such as human beings—is outside, in the cell's environment.

We know that the evolution of species on the earth has been highly dependent on environmental perturbations, including dramatic changes to landmasses, the gases in the air and water, and ambient temperature. These changes led to selection for new adaptive features in organisms, producing amazing diversity. As Darwin wrote in *On the Origin of Species* in 1859, "Owing to this struggle for life, any variation, however slight and from whatever cause proceeding, if it be in any degree profitable to an individual of any species, *in its infinitely complex relations to other organic beings and to external nature*, will tend to the preservation of that individual, and will generally be inherited by its offspring" (emphasis added). Darwin proposed that competition for limited resources would drive selection for individuals with traits that were best adapted to the environment. And when environments changed, so would these pressures, selecting for new traits that were better tuned to the new surroundings.

Similar Darwinian dynamics should apply to the evolution of cancers in our body. Even though we trained as a molecular biologist (DeGregori) and a physician (Gatenby), evolution and ecology have always fascinated both of us. Our extensive reading in these areas, while initially driven by what we thought was curiosity unrelated to our day jobs, revealed unappreciated parallels between the driving forces of evolution and our observations of cancer development and cancer patients' responses to therapy.

For instance, cancer researchers typically believed that a cancer-causing mutation would always confer an advantage to a cell that acquired it, but we recognized a classic evolutionary principle at work: A mutation does not automatically help or hinder an organism. Instead its effects are dependent on features of the local environment. In Darwin's finches, there is no "better" beak shape per se, but certain beaks improve survival under certain conditions. Similarly, we reasoned that a mutation that turns on a cancer-causing gene does not provide an inherent advantage to the cell and can, in fact, be disadvantageous if it makes that cell less able to use the resources of the tissue immediately around it.

We were also inspired by the punctuated equilibrium theory of paleontologists Niles Eldredge and Stephen Jay Gould, who noted that species often maintain stable traits through millions of years of fossil records, only to suddenly evolve rapidly in response to a dramatic environmental change. This concept stimulated our ideas about the way that some tissues could be initially unfavorable to cell mutations, but changes in those tissues, such as damage and inflammation in a smoker's lungs, could stimulate evolutionary change–sometimes leading to cancer.

We first saw this dynamic at work with aging-associated changes in bone marrow that led to the development of leukemias. Working with groups of young and old mice in DeGregori's Colorado lab, Curtis Henry, now at Emory University, and Andriy Marusyk, now at the Moffitt Cancer Center, created the same cancer-causing mutations in a few of the mice's bone marrow stem cells. The results showed that the same cancer-causing mutations can have very different effects on the fate of these cells, depending on age: the changes promoted the proliferation of mutated cells in the old mice but not in the young ones. And the determining factor did not appear to be in the mutated cells but in the metabolism and gene activity of the normal cells around them. For example, the activity of genes important for stem cell division and growth was reduced in nonmutated stem cells in the bone marrow of old mice, but it was restored in these cells when we introduced the cancer-causing mutation. Yet the mutation that helped these cells had bad effects on the mice. These stem cells normally generate key players in the body's immune system, but the population explosion of the cancer-mutated version of the cells instead led to the development of leukemias.

On the other hand, the fit young stem cells in the tissues of a young mouse already had levels of growth and energy use that nicely matched what their surroundings could provide. Therefore, such cells did not benefit from the cancer-causing mutations when we introduced them. The mutated cell populations did not grow. By favoring the status quo, youth is tumor-suppressive.

Why does any of this matter? Although we can avoid some mutations by not smoking and keeping clear of other mutagenic exposures, many, if not most, of the mutations that we accumulate in our cells during life cannot be dodged. But this new focus on tissue environments introduces a way to limit cancer: reversing tissue alterations caused by aging, smoking and other insults will reduce the success of cancer-causing mutations. The mutations will still occur, but they will be much less likely to give cells an advantage and thus will not grow in number.

Of course, there is no Fountain of Youth to reverse or prevent aging. Doing the things we know we should, such as exercising, eating a balanced diet and not smoking, can improve the maintenance of our tissues, which may be the best strategy we can use for the moment. But if we can figure out what key tissue environmental factors favor cancer development, we should be able to change these factors to limit malignancies. Indeed, in our mouse experiments, we showed that when we reduced the activity of inflammation-causing and tissue-damaging proteins in old mice, cells with the cancer-causing mutations did not proliferate; normal cells maintained their dominance. But we must proceed cautiously. Blocking inflammation in mice living in sterile cages may reduce cancer, but a similar strategy in people in the real world could limit defenses against infections because inflammation is part of our immune response.

From Prevention to Therapy

In addition to primary prevention, an evolutionary understanding can help make therapies for existing cancers more effective by reducing the nasty tendency of such cells to develop drug resistance. The evolution of resistance happens in other realms. Perhaps the most familiar example is the centuries-old contest between farmers and crop-destroying insects. For more than a century pesticide manufacturers produced a steady stream of new products, but the pests always evolved resistance. Eventually manufacturers recognized that trying to eradicate the pests by spraying high doses of pesticides on fields was making the problem worse because of an evolutionary process termed competitive release.

To understand competitive release, remember that all the insects within a large population occupying a field are continuously competing with one another for food and space, and they are not identical (as is also the case for cancer cells). In fact, for nearly every trait, including sensitivity to a pesticide, there is inevitable variability within a population. By spraying a large amount of insecticide (or administering a large dose of chemotherapy), the farmer (or oncologist) may kill the vast majority of insects (or cancer cells). Yet a few insects (or cells) have traits that make them less vulnerable, and with the highly vulnerable organisms removed, the resistant ones begin to spread. A farming strategy called integrated pest management tries to deal with this situation by using pesticides sparingly. Rather than trying to eradicate the pests, farmers spray only enough to control them and lower crop damage without resulting in competitive release. In this way, sensitivity of the pest to the pesticide is maintained.

The medical community has learned a similar lesson with antibiotics: excessive use must be stopped to curtail the constant evolutionary cycle that produces the development of drug-resistant pathogens. But this lesson has not yet taken hold in the cancer field.

Like farmers who used to blast fields with huge amounts of insecticides, doctors today typically give chemotherapy to patients at "maximum tolerated dose (MTD) until progression." Nearly all cancer drugs also damage normal tissues in the body, and these side effects can be very unpleasant and even fatal. MTD means the drugs are given in amounts that fall just short of killing the patient or causing intolerable side effects. Giving the same treatment "until progression" emerges from a traditional metric of treatment success, based on the tumor's change in size. Drugs are deemed successful when the tumor shrinks, and the treatment is abandoned if it gets bigger.

To most patients and doctors, treatment designed to kill the maximum number of cancer cells with relentless administration of the greatest possible amount of lethal drugs feels like the best approach. But as in the control of insects and infectious diseases, this strategy, in the setting of an incurable cancer, is often evolutionarily unwise because it sets in motion a series of events that actually accelerate the growth of drug-resistant cancer cells.

The other evolutionary lesson learned from pest control is that a "resistance management plan" can keep unwanted populations in check, often indefinitely. Can this strategy also lead to better outcomes for patients with incurable cancers? The answer is not yet clear, but there are hints from experimental studies and early clinical trials that it could do just that.

An evolution-based strategy for a patient who, after a month on an anticancer drug, had a 50 percent reduction in tumor size would be to stop treatment. This approach would be used only when we knew from past experience that available treatments–chemo, hormone therapy, surgery, immune system boosters–could not cure the cancer in this patient. Because a cure would not be achievable, the goal would instead be to keep the tumor from growing and metastasizing for as long as possible. By stopping therapy, we would leave behind a large number of treatment-sensitive cancer cells. The tumor would then begin to grow back and eventually reach its previous size. Yet during this regrowth period, because no chemotherapy would be administered, the majority of tumor cells would still be sensitive to the anticancer drug, not resistant to it. In effect, we would use the sensitive cells that we could control to suppress the growth of the resistant cells that we could not control. As a result, the treatment would be able to maintain tumor control much longer than the conventional approach of continuous administration of maximum dose and, because the drug dose would be significantly reduced, with much less toxicity and better quality of life.

Gatenby's lab began by investigating the approach in 2006 using mathematical models and computer simulations. Although such models had rarely been employed in cancer-treatment planning, the large number of possible treatment options required us to adopt an approach, common in physics, in which mathematical results help to define experimental methods that are likely to be successful. Our models defined the levels of drugs we wanted to test. The next step was to try those doses in mouse experiments, and doing so confirmed that tumor control could be greatly improved by evolution-based strategies.

The results were good enough to prompt a move into the clinic and a test on human cancer patients. We were joined in this effort by Jingsong Zhang, an oncologist at the Moffitt Cancer Center, who treats men with prostate cancer. With the help of Zhang, along with mathematicians and evolutionary biologists, we developed a model of the evolutionary dynamics of prostate cancer cells during treatment. We used this model to simulate the responses of prostate cancer to a variety of drug doses administered by an oncologist. Then we ran these encounters over and over again until we arrived at a series of doses that kept the cancer in check for the longest time without increasing the population of drug-resistant cells.

Next we asked patients with aggressive prostate cancer that had already metastasized to other locations—the kind that doctors cannot completely eliminate from the body—to volunteer for a clinical trial. So far the patients have had excellent outcomes. Of the 18 people enrolled, 11 are still in treatment. Standard therapy typically maintains control of metastatic prostate cancer for an average of about 13 months. In our trial, average tumor control is at least 34 months, and because more than half of our patients are still being treated actively, we cannot yet place an upper limit on how well they do. Furthermore, this control is being achieved using only 40 percent of the drug dose that patients would have received in standard treatment. But it is still early days for this treatment approach. Just because it works in prostate cancer does not mean it works in stomach cancer, for instance. And it may be tough to convince patients, even those with an incurable disease, that the best approach is not to kill as many cancer cells as possible but as few as necessary.

The Rules of Cancer

In many ways, the evolutionary model of cancer development and treatment serves to dispel the "mystery" of cancer. The proclivity of the disease to strike without any clear cause, along with its ability to overcome and return even after highly effective and often highly toxic therapy, can be viewed by patients and caregivers as both hopelessly complicated and magically powerful. In contrast, understanding that cancer obeys the rules of evolution like all other living systems can give us confidence that we have a chance to control it. Even without a cure, by using our understanding of evolutionary dynamics, we can strategically alter therapy to get the best possible outcome. And prevention strategies can be geared toward helping to create tissue landscapes in the body that favor normal cells over cancer cells.

For more than a century the cancer research community has sought "silver bullets"—drugs that can eliminate all cancer cells while sparing all normal cells. Cancer has been taking advantage of evolution to sidestep these drugs. But we can use evolution, too. We have the opportunity to expand the work of Darwin and his successors to develop more realistic approaches to both prevent and tame this deadly disease.

Referenced

Integrating Evolutionary Dynamics into Treatment of Metastatic Castrate-Resistant Prostate Cancer. Jingsong Zhang, Jessica J. Cunningham, Joel S. Brown and Robert A. Gatenby in *Nature Communications*, Vol. 8, Article No. 1816; November 28, 2017.

First Strike–Second Strike Strategies in Metastatic Cancer: Lessons from the Evolutionary Dynamics of Extinction. Robert A. Gatenby, Jingsong Zhang and Joel S. Brown in *Cancer Research* (in press).

About the Authors

James DeGregori is a professor of biochemistry and molecular genetics at the University of Colorado Anschutz Medical Campus and is author of Adaptive Oncogenesis: A New Understanding of How Cancer Evolves Inside Us *(Harvard University Press, 2018).*

Robert Gatenby is a physician and chair of the radiology department at the Moffitt Cancer Center in Tampa, Fla. He is also a member of the integrated mathematical oncology department there.

Section 5: Equity and Ethics in Cancer Care

We Must Improve Equity in Cancer Screening

By Melba Newsome

La Shawn Ford has always been meticulous about his health. He ate well, exercised regularly and never smoked. But last year, when the 48-year-old Illinois state representative learned that actor Chadwick Boseman had died of colon cancer, he decided to take his health-care game up a notch. In October 2020 Ford scheduled an appointment with his primary care physician for a colonoscopy and, while he was at it, a prostate cancer screening, too.

The colonoscopy came back clean, but his doctor refused to order the prostate-specific antigen (PSA) test, saying Ford wasn't in the recommended age range for screening. Although Ford had no indication that anything was amiss, he found another doctor to help him get the simple blood test.

Men with a PSA level between 4 and 10 have about a one-in-four chance of having prostate cancer. That risk goes to one in two if the level is above 10. Ford's was 11, so high that his physician ran the test again to confirm. This time it registered a PSA of 12.

Black men like Ford are disproportionately diagnosed with, and die from, prostate cancer, says Edward M. Schaeffer, chair of the urology department at the Northwestern Feinberg School of Medicine. "I'm surprised that if you're a Black man and you say to your doctor 'I want to get screened for prostate cancer because I'm at higher risk' that they would say no," he says. "That's kind of shocking to me, but I do see people like Representative Ford in my clinic not that infrequently."

Ford's subsequent blood work and MRI found further irregularities, and a biopsy confirmed that he had prostate cancer. Schaeffer performed a radical prostatectomy to remove Ford's entire prostate gland. Months later he was declared cancer-free.

"My cancer was already in an aggressive stage. It covered a lot of my prostate, but fortunately it was still contained," he says. "If

I had not advocated for myself and waited until I was 50, it could have been too late."

His experience illustrates two things: cancer screening can save lives, and cancer screening is not accessible for everyone who needs it. People of color, those of low wealth and residents of rural areas tend to be most vulnerable to screening disparities for reasons that are complex and often interrelated. Cost and lack of access, health illiteracy, implicit bias, and both cultural and structural barriers all play a role, as do disparities in cancer risk and vast differences in how screenings are integrated into patient care. The result is that too many cancers are detected too late, leading to too many avoidable deaths.

According to a report on cancer disparities from the American Association for Cancer Research, people of color receive significantly fewer recommended examinations than white people and are more likely to be diagnosed with advanced disease, lowering their chances of survival. "Cancer screening has huge inequities in this country," says Derek Raghavan, president of the Levine Cancer Institute in Charlotte, N.C. "The screening for breast, colon, prostate and lung cancer is way below what it should be in the African-American and Latino populations. If we could fix that, we could improve the death rate from cancer dramatically."

One Size Does Not Fit All

Medical societies and expert panels constantly reassess their screening guidelines in response to new research, using updated models and the most recent data. The result, however, may be confusing and seemingly inconsistent guidelines about who should be screened and how often, leaving many primary care providers unaware of the latest recommendations. It can mean huge variations in how these screenings are implemented–among both individual physicians and large health systems–as well as in how insurance companies reimburse for them. It can also mean huge variations in which patients receive the screenings they need.

Perhaps even more concerning, researchers such as Schaeffer say, is that medical groups often have homogeneous guidelines that do not account for variations among racial groups. With breast cancer, for instance, recent studies indicate that the incidence rate is higher in Black women younger than 45 and among white women older than 60. Yet the U.S. Preventive Services Task Force (USPSTF) and several other medical groups do not differentiate by race and recommend mammography screenings begin at age 50 for those at average risk. This does not acknowledge that Black women tend to have a more aggressive type of breast cancer that strikes at younger ages, argue researchers in a recent report in the *Journal of Breast Imaging*. For this group, those researchers recommend starting annual screening at age 40.

"The data surrounding the disparate incidence of breast cancer in Black women under 40 is compelling and must be considered as we look at cancer screening and diagnosis through the lens of health equity," says Monique Gary, chief medical adviser for Touch, the Black Breast Cancer Alliance and medical director of the cancer program at Grand View Health in Pennsylvania. "The current guidelines are an example of what happens when we 'don't see color.' They potentially place an already vulnerable group at significant risk for greater harm."

Similar disparities exist in cervical cancer. In 2018 both the USPSTF and the American Cancer Society (ACS) were recommending that women between the ages of 21 and 65 get a Pap smear every three years. Women between 30 and 65 were advised to have both a Pap and an hrHPV test, which screens for the presence of high-risk human papillomavirus–a major risk factor for cervical cancer–every three (ACS) to five (USPSTF) years. As though that weren't confusing enough, the ACS changed its stance in September 2020. Because cervical cancer is so rare in younger women, it suggested testing for hrHPV only and starting at age 25 rather than 21. The reasoning was that getting the more accurate HPV test every five years can reduce the risk of cervical cancer more effectively than a Pap test done every three.

That is troubling for some clinicians, who attribute disparities in cervical cancer incidence and mortality to lower access to screening. The incidence rate of cervical cancer among Hispanic women is 32 percent higher than for white women, and Black women are more likely to die of cervical cancer than any other racial or ethnic group. Limiting screening options could undermine cancer-prevention programs in vulnerable populations. If the new guidelines—which increase the suggested age of first screening—are widely adopted, insurers are likely to change reimbursements to match, something that could further decrease screening rates in the most underserved communities.

As Ford discovered last fall, screening guidelines strongly influence who gets referred for screening and what tests insurance providers will cover for whom. The trouble is that those guidelines are based on clinical trials conducted with subjects who are predominantly white.

Research shows that Black people are at a higher risk of lung cancer even if they smoke less over time, and their inclusion in clinical trials could have a significant impact on any screening guidelines that result. Raghavan points to the 2011 National Lung Cancer Screening trial, which studied more than 53,000 current or former heavy smokers to determine the cost and effectiveness of a form of screening called low-dose computed tomography (LDCT). Fewer than 5 percent of their participants were Black. A European trial on the same topic, the NELSON lung cancer study, also studied LDCT screening with 7,557 participants. The researchers made no mention of people of African ancestry.

Clinical trials investigating the benefits of prostate cancer screening also excluded Black men, despite greater incidence and mortality in this population. These trials, which consisted exclusively of white men, showed little or no benefit from PSA screening. As a result, in 2012 the USPSTF—concerned about overdiagnosis and treatment of small, benign or slow-growing cancers—recommended against using prostate cancer screening for anyone. The organization partially reversed its decision in 2018, recommending instead that for men age 55 to 69, screening decisions should be left up to the individual.

But some researchers are finally beginning to acknowledge the importance of diversity both in clinical trial participation and in establishing more relevant screening guidelines. A 2019 study in *JAMA Oncology* found that fewer Black smokers with lung cancer met the criteria for screening than white smokers with the disease. That is because Black smokers develop lung cancer at younger ages and at higher rates than white smokers. The researchers found that 68 percent of Black smokers were ineligible for screening at the time of their diagnosis, whereas 44 percent of white smokers were.

The USPSTF cited the study earlier this year as a factor in lowering its recommended screening age for lung cancer, from age 55 to 50, and reducing the number of pack years (years of smoking multiplied by the number of packs smoked per day) from 30 to 20, greatly expanding potential access. Nevertheless, only 5.7 percent of those at high risk are actually screened, in part because of the dearth of screening centers and lack of awareness.

The Cost Barrier

Improving access to, and awareness and affordability of, cancer screenings is what the Lung Bus was built to do. This 35-foot motor coach is the brainchild of the Levine Cancer Institute and is equipped with an LDCT scanner to serve people in local North Carolina communities with the highest risk of advanced lung cancer. These patients traditionally tend to have high rates of inoperable lung cancer, and they may also face transportation barriers or lack insurance.

Herbert Buff is one of them. Buff, 58, had smoked for more than 20 years but did not know it was possible to screen for lung cancer. In 2018 Buff went to the clinic in Morganton, N.C., for a routine doctor visit and casually mentioned that he sometimes had problems breathing. His doctor suggested a free screening on the Lung Bus. Buff's quick, noninvasive exam revealed a nickel-sized growth on his left lung that was later diagnosed as stage 1 lung cancer and was cured by surgery alone.

Since its first voyage in March 2017, the Lung Bus has achieved remarkable success in addressing health disparities. "We have used the bus exclusively to screen uninsured and underinsured people and the rural poor," says Raghavan, noting that they launched their screening program specifically to tackle the accessibility issues they saw in their patient population. They published the initial results in the *Oncologist* in 2020. "Our data show that of the 1,200 people we screened, 78 percent were rural poor and 20 percent were Black Americans. We found 30 lung cancers, of which 21 were at the potentially curable stage," he says. "You can overcome disparities of care if you really want to."

Cost factors into other screenings, too. The most advanced, accurate technologies for breast and cervical cancer screenings are more expensive and less accessible. Rural and underresourced areas are most likely to lag in getting the newest technology. Screening guidelines have long recommended HPV testing in conjunction with the Pap test, and randomized clinical trials have shown it results in better detection, fewer false positives and decreased mortality than Pap smears alone. But HPV testing is limited in the communities that have disproportionately high rates of cervical cancer incidence, morbidity and mortality.

Three-dimensional mammograms are another advance that has been more accessible to those with means, despite the fact that doctors say traditional mammograms are still the standard for all patients. The technology, which digitally sews numerous two-dimensional scans into a detailed 3-D image, can detect more cancers with fewer false positives than traditional mammography. But it's only selectively available. According to a study published in *JAMA Network Open*, Black and Latina women, as well as those who have less education and less income, have not been able to obtain 3-D mammography as easily as women who are white, are well educated or have a higher income. Clinics that serve these patients simply do not have the necessary tools. "[The] equipment is more expensive, and it's not available everywhere," says Diana

Dickson-Witmer, a breast surgeon and head of the BeeBe Center for Breast Health in Rehoboth Beach, Del.

Structural and Cultural Barriers

In the decade since the passage of the Affordable Care Act in 2010, more Americans than ever have gained access to health insurance. Expanded government coverage has gone a long way toward making cancer-screening access more equitable by eliminating many out-of-pocket costs, according to research by the ACS. As just one example, a report in the *Journal of Cancer* in July 2020 found that U.S. states that expanded Medicaid had fewer men with high PSA results, indicating they were getting screened earlier than those living in states that had not expanded Medicaid. In this case, at least, insurance appeared directly correlated to better screening outcomes.

Addressing cost is a good start, says Tomi Akinyemiju, a cancer epidemiologist and associate director for community outreach and engagement at the Duke Cancer Institute. Akinyemiju explores the interconnection of race, ethnicity, income and access to health care and develops outreach strategies for communities in North Carolina. "People in Black, Hispanic or Latinx communities are less likely to have received the screening that they are eligible for," she says. "Affordability ... is a big reason, especially for minorities and those of low income, but there are also other really important dimensions separate from the cost."

Eliminating screening disparities requires tackling structural barriers, Akinyemiju says. These can include knowing the location of the nearest facility, being able to get there and setting up hours that accommodate people with inflexible work schedules.

Education–of risk factors and, consequently, what screening is needed and when–is yet another structural issue. Many people lack basic understanding or a primary care provider to help inform them. When Tanya Weaver, an independent community health advocate, began working to get breast cancer screenings for underserved Black women in Portsmouth, Va., more than a decade ago, many did not even understand what care they needed or whom they should contact for information.

"Many of the women couldn't even pronounce the word 'mammogram,' and some confused mammograms with having breast cancer because no one had educated them," Weaver says. "When the city sent out informational pamphlets, they were all earmarked for the more affluent areas of Portsmouth."

Even once someone gets past all that, Akinyemiju says, interactions with providers are vital, too. "Do they talk down to you? Do they explain things in language that is easy to understand? Do they answer your questions respectfully and show concern and care for you?" If not, she says, then patients are far less likely to return for future screenings.

That is precisely what Weaver has seen with the women she works with. She arranged free mammograms for them at a local hospital, never imagining they would be derided for taking care of their health. "Many of the women came back dejected and said they would never go back because they felt like they weren't wanted there," Weaver says. "They overheard one person say, 'They keep coming in here with these coupons to get a free mammogram.'"

Today there is growing evidence–medical, epidemiological and sociological–that cancer-related disparities are closely linked to extensive influences known as social determinants of health, which involve the conditions in which people live and work that affect their health risks and outcomes. There is also a growing understanding by clinicians and other health-care providers that helping those most affected will require focused and coordinated social action. Academic institutions and health-care systems around the country are building multidisciplinary programs that prioritize health equity so that the most vulnerable people get the cancer screening tests they need.

One of those programs is at Northwestern, where Ford received his care. Northwestern Medicine's Project HOPE (Health Outreach Promoting Equity) educates local communities in the Chicago area about health disparities, aiming to increase equity in health outcomes. During primary care screenings, doctors now routinely talk with their patients about how they are doing financially and socially. They ask them to describe their living conditions to better understand and address any underlying issues. Ford, now a vocal proponent of regular health checks and of being one's own medical advocate, works with Project HOPE to reach others in situations similar to his.

Today Project HOPE and other programs are identifying ways to help close the cancer-equity gap, in screening and beyond. Patients who have good information, who are treated with respect and kindness, and who have people to help guide them through a confounding process are able to make better decisions, Schaeffer says. "By beginning to identify these different social determinants of health, we can impact this and make a difference," he says. "There are glimmers of hope for continued progress."

This article is part of "Innovations In: Cancer Early Detection," an editorially independent special report that was produced with financial support from Johnson & Johnson.

About the Author

Melba Newsome is an award-winning science, health and environmental reporter. She lives in Charlotte, N.C.

The Race to Stop a Plastics Plant Scores a Crucial Win

By Judith Enck, Rebekah Creshkoff

As an old saying goes, you can't fight city hall, meaning government. But the people of St. James Parish, La., did just that—and they won a major court victory against a massive plastics plant supported by the governor, state and local legislators, the business community and local power brokers.

Led by Sharon Lavigne of Rise St. James, a faith-based grassroots organization fighting to reduce pollution in the community, and lawyers at Earthjustice, a national nonprofit environmental law organization, and other community groups led the years-long battle. Ultimately, the groups persuaded Louisiana's 19th Judicial District Court to cancel 14 air pollution permits granted by the state's Department of Environmental Quality that would have allowed Formosa Plastics to build its proposed petrochemical complex. Petrochemicals are in a slew of products, including plastics.

This project would have created the largest plastics plant in the world and subjected the residents of St. James Parish to another 800 tons of hazardous air pollutants every year—on top of the air pollution they already breathe from miles and miles of refineries and other petrochemical facilities that dot the landscape.

This stunning legal decision is just a single case, and the company has promised to appeal. But, as the head of an organization with environmental policy expertise, we believe the win will galvanize equally effective local opposition in other places across the country where similar facilities are being proposed—invariably in low-income communities of color, primarily in Texas, Louisiana and the areas that make up Appalachia.

Meanwhile, the world is already overflowing with single-use plastic, most of which is neither recyclable nor biodegradable. The decision will also prevent additional carbon pollution from being spewed into the atmosphere when the nation urgently needs to slow climate change by reducing greenhouse gas emissions.

As investments in renewable energy and electric vehicles cause demand for fossil fuels to decline, the oil and gas industry is turning to plastics to keep making money.

This trend has alarming implications for the climate crisis. Last October, a report from our organization, Beyond Plastics, found that greenhouse gas emissions from plastics production in the United States are on track to outpace domestic coal emissions by 2030. The Formosa project alone would have emitted more than 13.6 million tons of greenhouse gases a year—equivalent to what 3.5 coal-fired power plants would emit in the same year.

But stopping, or at least slowing, Formosa's project is just part of reducing the overall pollution burden for St. James Parish, which is located along an 85-mile stretch of the Mississippi River between Baton Rouge and New Orleans known as "Cancer Alley." The corridor, in which many low-income people live, houses about 150 petrochemical plants and refineries, and the risk that people of color living nearby will develop cancer over the course of their lifetime is significantly higher than the national average.

According to their permit application, Formosa Plastics' project would have doubled or even tripled the levels of carcinogens St. James residents breathe. Twelve petrochemical facilities are already within a 10-mile radius of the site where Formosa wants to build, and the new complex would make the concentration of pollution even worse than it is today.

The company's own modeling, part of their permit application, showed that inhaling the excessive concentrations of soot and nitrogen dioxide emitted at the facility could cause such disorders as asthma and chronic obstructive pulmonary disease (COPD). Yet Formosa callously proposed to build this noxious complex just a mile away from an elementary school.

Plans for the 2,400-acre complex included 10 chemical plants, key among them two enormous "ethane crackers." In such facilities, hydrofracked gases are superheated until the molecules "crack" into smaller hydrocarbons, particularly ethylene, which is then transformed into plastic pellets. The pellets are used to make plastic bags, plastic bottles, plastic straws and other consumer items–many to be used just once, then persisting in the environment for decades.

This attempted expansion of petrochemical facilities in Louisiana, Texas and Appalachia is creating "sacrifice zones" where big companies believe local residents are just as disposable as the plastic they manufacture.

While existing ethane crackers are already operating, all eyes are on communities where fights similar to the one with Formosa are unfolding–and where opponents of planned facilities are now energized by this legal victory.

Most notably, Shell has built the nation's newest ethane cracker in the tiny community of Potter Township, Pa., on the Ohio River. That plastic production facility is expected to start operating any day now. Residents and environmental groups are concerned that it will attract other mega-polluters to the area, creating large-scale pollution problems, making it a northern version of Cancer Alley in the Ohio River Valley.

These companies are forcing residents to pay with their health, and to what end? So that consumers don't need to bring a reusable bag to the store or drink from a durable coffee cup?

In Louisiana, state and company officials claim the Formosa complex would create 1,200 jobs and add millions of dollars to the local economy. But there are more environmentally sustainable ways to create jobs that do not damage the health of workers, their communities and the planet.

If this court decision is reversed upon appeal, Formosa might still be allowed to build. But Louisiana and other states need to stop falling for the jobs-versus-environment argument. Climate disasters around the world make it apparent that we need to rapidly slash greenhouse gas emissions and that transitioning away from fossil fuels will create jobs.

The time for Louisiana to change direction is now, as the federal government is poised to pump significant new funding into renewable energy projects. Yet, if we just switch to renewable energy sources while continuing to manufacture ever-increasing amounts of plastic, we are guaranteed to rocket past the crucial 1.5-degree Celsius climate threshold, which will result in more severe heat waves, greater sea-level rise, more flooding, reduced agricultural output and more extreme weather all over the globe.

This is the moment for those in government and business to rethink their antiquated economic development strategies, which should be based on providing living-wage jobs that do not threaten public health. We can't create any more sacrifice zones.

A judge has spoken, but the courts are not the only segment of government with a responsibility to the health and environmental welfare of our communities. Congress needs to put a pause on the race to construct more petrochemical facilities. We cannot allow these investments to lock us into a future framed by plastic and all the problems it creates, in terms of human, ecosystem and planetary health.

This is an opinion and analysis article, and the views expressed by the author or authors are not necessarily those of Scientific American.

About the Authors

Judith Enck is a former Environmental Protection Agency regional administrator and currently is a visiting professor at Bennington College and president of Beyond Plastics.

Rebekah Creshkoff is a volunteer with Beyond Plastics.

Clinical Trials Have the Best Medicine but Do Not Enroll the Patients Who Need It

By David H. Freedman

Jean Reimers, a 75-year-old retired supermarket cashier, enjoys her life in Grand Island, Neb., a small city near the Platte River that boasts attractions such as the Stuhr Museum of the Prairie Pioneer and a sandhill crane nature reserve. Nearly two years ago Reimers found out from her local doctor that she had cancer. The worse news was that it was late-stage metastatic lung cancer, hard to treat and with a dismally low survival rate. The standard approach in such cases is palliative care to keep dying patients comfortable. "It looked like I probably wouldn't be around another year," she says.

Today not only is Reimers still around, but she says she feels great. She has lots of energy and no pain. This past fall CT scans showed all her tumors have shrunk or disappeared entirely. And she was anticipating the birth of her 11th grandchild. "I've got a lot of things I still want to do," she says.

Her high-quality time, Reimers says, comes thanks to experimental drugs she received as part of a clinical trial. The treatment, a combination of two immunotherapies called ipilimumab and nivolumab, is not yet approved for lung cancer by the U.S. Food and Drug Administration. The trial Reimers took part in was one of the tests to see if the regimen works.

This would not be an unusual story if Reimers was a patient at a big-name, big-city academic medical center. The very top cancer hospitals, such as the University of Texas MD Anderson Cancer Center in Houston and New York City's Memorial Sloan Kettering Cancer Center, enroll about 25 percent of their patients in trials. But Reimers, like Grand Island's other 51,000 residents, lives closest to CHI Health St. Francis, a typical small community hospital that is part of a regional network but has no formal ties to any major medical institution. "I didn't think people in small towns had the same chances for trials that people in big cities do," Reimers says. Her only option, she thought, was to drive nearly three hours every two weeks to a bigger hospital in Omaha. She would likely have had to stay overnight instead of going straight home to rest, and she probably would not have done it. But the head oncologist at St. Francis's cancer treatment center found out that Reimers met the criteria for the double-drug trial, filled out the forms, followed up and got her in.

The drugs available in clinical trials often represent the latest in research, and many turn out to be significantly more effective than standard treatments. Half of all drugs that make it into the last of three phases of drug trials, when most patients enter those trials, end up being approved by the FDA because of these improved results. The drug Herceptin, for instance, was only available in trials before it became a mainline treatment for breast cancer in 1998 and since then has been prescribed to 420,000 women. More recently, some 90,000 breast cancer patients have been treated with Ibrance, but before 2015 the drug was given only in trials. Another medication, Keytruda, was approved after clinical trials in 2014; now some 70,000 patients with a number of different types of cancer have used it.

But whereas about one third of cancer patients in the U.S. meet the criteria for a trial with a new drug, only about 4 percent end up in such tests, according to National Cancer Institute estimates, and some experts say the real number is even lower. The main reason for the massive shortfall: in the nonacademic community hospitals where most cancer patients are treated, doctors do not feel they have the time, the incentives or the support to learn about available trials, to qualify and enroll patients, or to provide the extra follow-up care such trials often call for. A National Academies of Sciences, Engineering, and Medicine study concluded that "community practitioners lack the needed infrastructure and support to actively participate in clinical trials." A study in the clinical cancer journal CA called trial enrollment "embarrassingly low" and blamed it, in part, on "a lack of knowledge about available studies by community oncologists, a lack of time or interest, or a lack of resources to support the cost of performing clinical trials." Because nationally about 85 percent of cancer patients end up at community hospitals, most of the low participation in cancer trials is attributable to the failure of those hospitals to enroll their patients.

Low trial enrollment, which effectively cuts patients off from lifesaving medicine, is a giant national health problem. For example, fewer than 1 percent of patients who have Alzheimer's disease enter a trial. But for cancer, the missed opportunities are especially painful, experts say, because drug development in this area has been particularly strong. "Many of our drug trials involve the most promising agents we've seen," says Tufia Haddad, an oncology researcher at the Mayo Clinic. Thanks to new ways of identifying and targeting mutations in tumors and to immunotherapies that help muster the body's natural defenses against cancers, there are more than 600 experimental cancer drugs that have shown good results in animals and in early small studies in humans. And contrary to common belief, patients in the vast majority of cancer drug trials do not risk getting a placebo–these trials test the best standard treatment against a new medication.

The enrollment problem also handicaps research. Lack of patients forces many trials to stop before getting results, ending the progress of many promising treatments. Most trials are at least delayed by patient enrollment shortages. About one out of six of all trials never manage to recruit a single patient. "The biggest problem in developing new drugs is a lack of patients to treat with them," says John T. Cole, an oncologist at the Ochsner Health System based in New Orleans, who oversees a network of oncology practices. "We can't meet that challenge unless we solve the problem of low enrollment in community hospitals."

Politicians and regulators have done little to help community hospitals and doctors surmount the obstacles, according to R. Alta Charo, a law professor at the University of Wisconsin–Madison, who studies medical research policy. Instead they have passed "right to try" legislation, which prohibits the FDA from denying terminal patients access to experimental drugs that are not available to them in clinical trials. In fact, the FDA almost never denies such access, so the law is unlikely to help more than a handful of patients and does nothing to improve access to clinical trials. "Helping overwhelmed and underresourced doctors at community hospitals would be a much better approach," Charo says.

Finding effective ways to help, however, is not easy. There are partial solutions, such as artificial-intelligence programs that crunch through reams of data to match patients to trials. Other attempted remedies are low tech and involve a range of outreach, education and marketing tools that can change the antitrial culture of community hospitals. To succeed, however, these approaches need to help doctors cope with the time constraints, lack of expertise and financial obstacles that keep them from getting patients into trials. St. Francis, which shares those small hospital disadvantages, manages to place some 35 percent of its cancer patients in trials. That achievement is due almost entirely to the determination and dedication of Mehmet Copur, the head oncologist at the time of Reimers's treatment. But counting on every other community hospital to display the same fervor is a risky gamble.

One Doctor's Mission

When Reimers became ill, Copur was willing to put in the extra work required to find out about appropriate trials and get her into one–work built into the infrastructure of academic centers but not community hospitals–just as he has been doing for his other patients. To refuse to go that extra mile is to fail to provide seriously ill patients with their best possible prospects, insists Copur, who recently moved to the Morrison Cancer Center in the nearby community of Hastings, where he is building a similar clinical trial program. "The standard of care today is what was in trials 10 years ago," he says. "To put patients in a trial is to give them a chance to get a drug that will be the standard of care 10 years from now."

In 1995 Copur was a young medical scientist from Turkey doing basic research at the National Institutes of Health outside of

Washington, D.C., when a change in government policy—an alteration in temporary work permit numbers—suddenly left him in imminent danger of losing his visa. His only hope for staying in the U.S. was a program that grants permanent visas to doctors who spend three years treating patients in an underserved community. He saw a listing for a job at Grand Island's St. Francis. Copur grabbed the position.

"But when I got here I said to myself, 'My God, my career is over,'" he recalls. Copur had intended to continue some clinical research in the job, but he found that St. Francis had no medical library and no Internet access at the time. Clinical trials were almost nonexistent, and when Copur proposed that he at least try to participate in some, neither his fellow oncologists nor the hospital administration seemed open to the idea. "It was a fight from the beginning," he says. "Even in big-city hospitals people don't always see how important clinical trials are, let alone a small-town hospital."

The problem was that to earn his salary Copur had to see a stream of patients, five days a week. But clinical trials require extra work, with each patient taking up on average about three times as much time as a nontrial patient, thanks to extra record keeping and close patient-monitoring requirements. In academic centers, doctors are given that extra time and can draw on a trial-focused support staff. Copur had to do it all on his own, including establishing rigorous data collection, performing extra diagnostic tests, conducting extra patient visits, producing reports, training staff, and more. He also brought in funding from the NCI and joined a research consortium of hospitals that made more trials available.

Many of his patients hesitated to join a trial, saying they did not want to be guinea pigs who might end up with a highly toxic drug or a placebo—widely held misconceptions that are particularly common among rural patients, says James Atkins, an oncologist at the Southeastern Medical Oncology Center in North Carolina. Copur patiently explained to them that cancer trials today are designed with patient benefit in mind and that the worst case was usually getting the drug they would have received anyway. Most of his patients consented. Then other oncologists at St. Francis started to notice that Copur's trial patients sometimes did surprisingly well. Of course they were doing well, Copur explained: some of them were receiving much better drugs. Soon his colleagues began looking for trials for their own patients.

"Copur has done a great job in a completely rural environment," says Praveen Vikas, an oncologist at the University of Iowa Health Care. "He's that rare kind of community physician who can provide the kind of care that often beats physicians in academic settings in terms of value and patient satisfaction, while staying on top of research."

As of 2018, Copur's team at St. Francis had enrolled patients in 74 different trials. But to do so, Copur worked nonstop from dawn, taking off one hour at 7 P.M. to have dinner at home with his ailing father before returning to spend another three hours at the clinic. "These trials are my whole life," he says. "Sometimes I dream about making that big fundamental research contribution, but then my patients remind me that what I am doing here is a bigger contribution."

One of those patients is a young man (he asked not to be identified) who learned two years ago that his kidney cancer was spreading. Approved chemotherapies did not offer much hope, so he started searching out clinical trials, assuming he would have to go far from his home near Grand Island to get in one. He traveled to Washington, D.C., to meet with a specialist–who told him to get right back to Nebraska and see Copur. "To be honest, I was a little skeptical when I met Dr. Copur, and he told me he'd get me in the right trial," he recalls. "But my phone started pinging with e-mails about trials by the time I was pulling out of the parking lot." Today the patient is thriving and credits the immunotherapy drugs he received through the trial that Copur enrolled him in.

Breaking Barriers

Copur's experience at St. Francis proves that community hospitals can succeed as clinical trial centers. And if he can deliver on his quest to duplicate that success at the even smaller Morrison Cancer

Center, which is part of the Mary Lanning Healthcare community hospital in Hastings, the evidence will be all the more impressive. Community hospitals do not need to hit 35 percent enrollment, as St. Francis has, to make a big dent in the trial gap. If only one fourth of community hospitals boosted their trial enrollment to an average of 10 percent, it would result in an increase of 50 percent in the number of cancer patients enrolled in trials. In a survey of a wide range of cancer patients, 81 percent reported their doctors did not discuss the possibility of trials with them. In a separate survey of women with cancer, more than half reported that their oncologists either did not mention trials or even actively discouraged patients from participating in one.

The St. Francis work also highlights the obstacles that community hospitals face. But a 10 percent gain in enrollment does not require daunting personal sacrifice, say clinicians who have helped other community hospitals make the jump. Atkins, who directs a large clinical trial consortium across the southeastern U.S., is working with 25 hospitals in five states to help them boost clinical trial enrollment. Many physicians have gotten onboard, Atkins says. It means going beyond the typical physician's 50-or-so-hour week but only by five hours or less. "It's extra work for doctors, but if a doctor doesn't want to do it for patients, that seems a little lazy to me," he says.

Clinical trials can also be redesigned to reduce the burden on community hospital physicians, shifting more of the workload to the research centers that originate the trials. A study led by the University of Pittsburgh Medical Center, along with six other academic medical centers and the National Institutes of Health, looked at 38 steps that clinical trial leaders can take to get more doctors at other hospitals involved in their trials, steps mostly aimed at raising doctors' interest while reducing the workload involved in opening the trial and in enrolling patients. The steps included sending researchers out to hospitals to speak to staff about the trial's relevance, the benefits to patients and the patients' qualifications; providing follow-up teleconference meetings; writing articles for the hospital newsletter and for local and physician publications;

establishing 24/7 access for researchers to get questions answered; putting up a Web site dedicated to the trial; and making available patient-recruitment aids such as multilingual brochures and consent forms. The study, published in 2014 in *Clinical Pediatrics*, found there was a 38 percent jump in recruitment after the steps were taken.

Sonika Bhatnagar, lead author and an associate professor of pediatrics at the University of Pittsburgh School of Medicine, notes that some factors stood out during the study. "The biggest physician barrier was time constraints," she says. "Minimizing their workload was critical, and we found making everything as simple as possible made a big difference." Among the aids Bhatnagar and her colleagues provided physicians were prepackaged talking points to use with patients, so the doctors did not have to study a trial's methodology in detail to explain it accurately. The researchers also offered to reach out directly to a patient's family to address their concerns. And physicians worry that putting a patient in a trial will compromise his or her autonomy in making care decisions, Bhatnagar adds, because trials often tightly circumscribe some treatment options. She has found that the best way to counter that concern is for researchers to go to hospitals to meet as many physicians as possible in person to build trust in the trial's protocol and to create enthusiasm about what the trial might do both for individual patients and for the countless patients everywhere who might ultimately be helped by the trial's findings. "Most physicians would take a lot of pride in contributing to research that could ultimately change treatment guidelines for the field," Bhatnagar says.

Another study gave doctors materials designed to streamline the process of patient screening–that is, determining which patients qualify–and to make it easier to follow trial protocols during treatment. The study also involved adding one-on-one meetings between local physicians and trial researchers and on-site discussions about the disease being treated. In that study, enrollment at the targeted facilities more than doubled.

Some trial outreach efforts are being facilitated by the fact that academic medical centers are looking to expand in their states, and sometimes beyond, via acquiring or partnering with community hospitals. Existing big health networks are also pushing outreach. Kaiser Permanente—a nonprofit health care company—has nudged and supported all its 27 northern California hospitals, many of them community hospitals, into enrolling cancer patients into trials. "Instead of having to drive 50 miles or more to an academic medical center, our patients can be treated in a clinical trial in the same place they delivered their babies and got their flu shots," says Lou Fehrenbacher, a Kaiser Permanente oncologist who oversees the region's cancer trials program. Likewise Yale University's main hospital, based in New Haven, has been bringing in affiliated community oncology clinics around Connecticut into clinical studies. Unfortunately, most of the nation's 4,000 community hospitals are not closely allied with an academic center, so this approach may be limited.

The High-Tech Fix

It may be, though, that technology can help close that particular gap. The Mayo Clinic has been testing a pilot of an ambitious approach, based on IBM's Watson cognitive-computing platform. That system has been looking at all the details in the records of every breast cancer patient at the medical center and matching them against the 16 different clinical trials for breast cancer available there. The Mayo claims that after 11 months the system was able to increase combined enrollment in those trials by 80 percent—though so far only at the clinic itself and not yet at community hospitals. According to the Mayo's Haddad, who is helping to run the pilot, the big jump is owed in part to the fact that the project included increased staffing and focus around patient-trial matching. But she adds that Watson's ability to zip through not only tightly specified data fields in the health records but also clinical notes and other unstructured data has made a big difference in the system's hit rate. "Most electronic health record systems aren't sophisticated enough to be able to answer questions such as which treatments the patient has already had," she says. "More than 90 percent of the data in records is in unstructured form, and cognitive systems can go after it."

A study run by the NCI and Case Western Reserve University, using another experimental cognitive-computing-based system called Trial Prospector, scoured the records of 60 new gastrointestinal cancer patients across several clinics and matched 57 percent of them to at least one of 15 different trials. A group of oncologists brought into the study gave the system a big thumbs-up, deeming all the matches to be accurate. Another system tested at Cincinnati Children's Hospital Medical Center was found to reduce the time needed to match patients to trials by 85 percent.

Exciting results, but they come with serious qualifications. For one thing, such systems generally require that a hospital have a sophisticated electronic health record system in place to feed them data. Most community hospitals currently have systems that are too rudimentary to allow programming in trial-matching capabilities. But given medicine's growing reliance on mining electronic health records for advancing patient care, those systems will inevitably be upgraded to the point where automating trial matching will become feasible–especially as more community hospitals become affiliated with larger hospitals and even academic medical centers.

Copur, for his part, maintains that what will ultimately bring clinical trial options to that great majority of cancer patients will be a slowly growing wave of peer pressure as more clinicians in community settings start to see the light. Copur himself keeps publishing–63 papers and articles to date, such as a study in the *Journal of Clinical Oncology* evaluating treatments for metastatic pancreatic cancer–and giving talks about what a community hospital can accomplish. "I tell doctors that if they're not looking for ways to put their patients in clinical trials, they should be referring them to a doctor who will," he says.

What seems poised to effect change, if slowly, is a combination of all those approaches: Trial researchers who get out into communities and market their work to local doctors, trial designs that reduce physician workload, and tools that automate patient-trial matching and related tasks. It will also take strong advocates like Copur and the NCI willing to sound a constant, loud drumbeat that links trials to the duty that all physicians—not just those in academia—have to the profession and to their patients. It will only be then, if those efforts on multiple fronts put more people in trials, that patients win the real right to try.

Referenced

Clinical Trial Awareness, Attitudes, and Participation among Patients with Cancer and Oncologists. Laurie Fenton et al. in *Community Oncology*, Vol. 6, No. 5, pages 207–213; May 2009.

Transforming Clinical Research in the United States: Challenges and Opportunities: Workshop Summary. Institute of Medicine. National Academies Press, 2010.

Reliability of Adverse Symptom Event Reporting by Clinicians. Thomas M. Atkinson et al. in *Quality of Life Research*, Vol. 21, No. 7, pages 1159–1164; September 2012.

Alzheimer's Disease Drug Development Pipeline: 2017. Jeffrey Cummings et al. in Alzheimer's & Dementia: Translational Research & *Clinical Interventions*, Vol. 3, No. 3, pages 367–384; September 2017.

About the Author

David H. Freedman is a journalist who has been covering science, business and technology for more than 30 years.

The Cancer Industry: Hype vs. Reality

By John Horgan

First, some basic facts to convey the scale of the problem. Cancer is the second most lethal disease in the U.S., behind only heart disease. More than 1.7 million Americans were diagnosed with cancer in 2018, and more than 600,000 died. Over 15 million Americans cancer survivors are alive today. Almost four out of ten people will be diagnosed in their lifetime, according to the National Cancer Institute.

Cancer has spawned a huge industrial complex involving government agencies, pharmaceutical and biomedical firms, hospitals and clinics, universities, professional societies, nonprofit foundations and media. The costs of cancer care have surged 40 percent in the last decade, from $125 billion in 2010 to $175 billion in 2020 (projected).

Research funding has also surged. The budget of the National Cancer Institute, a federal agency founded in 1937, now totals over $6 billion/year. That is a fraction of the total spent on research by nonprofit foundations ($6 billion a year, according to 2019 study), private firms and other government agencies. Total research spending since Richard Nixon declared a "war on cancer" in 1971 exceeds a quarter trillion dollars, according to a 2016 estimate.

Cancer-industry boosters claim that investments in research, testing and treatment have led to "incredible progress" and millions of "cancer deaths averted," as the homepage of the American Cancer Society, a nonprofit that receives money from biomedical firms, puts it. A 2016 study found that cancer experts and the media often describe new treatments with terms such as "breakthrough," "game changer," "miracle," "cure," "home run," "revolutionary," "transformative," "life saver," "groundbreaking" and "marvel."

There are more than 1,200 accredited cancer centers in the U.S. They spent $173 million on television and magazine ads directed at the public in 2014, according to a 2018 study, and 43 of the 48 top spenders "deceptively promot[ed] atypical patient experiences through the use of powerful testimonials." A 2014 study concluded that cancer centers "frequently promote cancer therapy with emotional appeals that evoke hope and fear while rarely providing information about risks, benefits, costs, or insurance availability."

Little Net Progress After 90 Years, Besides Anti-Smoking Efforts

What's the reality behind the hype? "No one is winning the war on cancer," Azra Raza, an oncologist at Columbia, asserts in her 2019 book *The First Cell: And the Costs of Pursuing Cancer to the Last*. Claims of progress are "mostly hype, the same rhetoric from the same self-important voices for the past half century." Trials have yielded improved treatments for childhood cancers and specific cancers of the blood, bone-marrow and lymph systems, Raza notes. But these successes, which involve uncommon cancers, are exceptions among a "litany of failures."

The best way to measure progress against cancer is to look at mortality rates, the number of people who succumb to cancer per unit of population per year. The risk of cancer grows with age. (Although childhood cancer gets a lot of attention, Americans under 20 years old account for less than 0.3 percent of all U.S. cancer deaths.) Hence as the average life span of a population grows (because of advances against heart and respiratory disorders, infectious disease and so on), so does the cancer mortality rate. To calculate mortality trends over time, therefore, researchers adjust for the aging of the population.

With this adjustment–which, keep in mind, presents cancer medicine in a more favorable light–mortality rates have declined almost 30 percent since 1991. This trend, according to cancer-industry boosters, shows that investments in research, tests and treatments have paid off. What boosters often fail to mention is that recent declines in cancer mortality follow at least 60 years of increases. The current age-adjusted mortality rate for all cancers in the U.S., 152.4 deaths per 100,000 people, is just under what it was in 1930, according to a recent analysis.

The rise and fall of cancer deaths track the rise and fall of smoking, with a lag of a couple of decades. Cigarette consumption in the U.S. more than doubled between 1930 and the early 1970s and has fallen steadily since then, according to the nonprofit site Our World in Data. Smoking raises the risk of many cancers but especially of lung cancer, which is by far the biggest killer, accounting for more deaths than colon, breast and prostate cancer combined.

Over the past two decades lung-cancer mortality has dropped, but it still remains higher than it was in the 1960s, especially among women, according to Our World in Data. A 2006 analysis concluded that without reductions in smoking "there would have been virtually no reduction in overall cancer mortality in either men or women since the early 1990s."

New Treatments Yield Small Benefits, Big Costs

Research has linked cancer to many internal and external factors, notably oncogenes, hormones, viruses, carcinogens (such as those in cigarettes) and random cellular replication errors, or "bad luck." But with the notable exception of the smoking/cancer link, which led to effective anti-smoking measures, that knowledge has not translated into significantly improved preventive measures or treatments. Clinical cancer trials "have the highest failure rate compared with other therapeutic areas," according to a 2012 paper.

Pharmaceutical companies keep bringing new drugs to market. But one study found that 72 new anticancer drugs approved by the FDA between 2004 and 2014 prolonged survival for an average of 2.1 months. A 2017 report concluded that "most cancer drug approvals have not been shown to, or do not, improve clinically relevant end points," including survival and quality of life. The authors worried that "the FDA may be approving many costly, toxic drugs that do not improve overall survival."

Costs of cancer treatments have vastly outpaced inflation, and new drugs are estimated to cost on average more than $100,000/year. Patients end up bearing a significant proportion of costs. More than 40 percent of people diagnosed with cancer lose their life savings within 2 years, according to one estimate.

Immune therapies, which seek to stimulate immune responses to cancer, have generated enormous excitement. Two researchers won the 2018 Nobel Prize for work related to immune therapies, and a new book, *The Breakthrough: Immunotherapy and the Race to Cure Cancer*, claims that they represent a "revolutionary discovery in our understanding of cancer and how to beat it."

According to a 2018 report in *Stat News*, drug firms aggressively market immune therapies, and patients are "pushing hard to try them, even when there is little to no evidence the drugs will work for their particular cancer." A 2017 analysis by oncologists Nathan Gay and Vinay Prasad estimated that fewer than 10 percent of cancer patients can benefit from immune therapies, and that is a "best-case scenario."

Immune therapies trigger severe side effects, and they are also extremely expensive, costing hundreds of thousands of dollars a year, oncologist Siddhartha Mukherjee, author of *The Emperor of All Maladies*, a bestselling history of cancer, reported in the *New Yorker* last year. "Subsequent hospital stays and supportive care can drive the total costs to a million dollars or more," he writes. If widely prescribed, immune therapies "could bankrupt the American health-care system."

Tests Lead to Overdiagnosis and Overtreatment

The cancer industry, aided by celebrities who claim that tests saved their lives, has convinced the public that screening for cancer is beneficial. The earlier we can detect cancerous cells, the more likely it is that treatment will succeed. Right? Wrong. One of the most significant findings of the past decade is that many people have cancerous or pre-cancerous cells that, if left untreated, would never have compromised their health. Autopsies have revealed that many people who die of unrelated causes harbor cancerous tissue.

Tests cannot reliably distinguish between harmful and harmless cancers. As a result, widespread testing has led to widespread overdiagnosis, the flagging of non-harmful cancerous cells. Overdiagnosis leads in turn to unnecessary chemotherapy, radiation and surgery. Gilbert Welch, a physician whose 2011 book *Overdiagnosed: Making People Sick in Pursuit of Health* helped bring overdiagnosis to light, recently called it "an unfortunate side effect of our irrational exuberance for early detection." Overdiagnosis is more insidious than false positives, when tests erroneously indicate the presence of cancer. Biopsies can overturn false positives but not overdiagnoses.

Mammograms and prostate-specific antigen (PSA) tests have led to especially high rates of overdiagnosis and overtreatment for breast and prostate cancer. A 2013 meta-analysis by the Cochrane Collaboration, an international association of experts that assesses medical procedures, estimated that if 2,000 women have mammograms over a period of 10 years, one woman's life will be saved by a positive diagnosis. Meanwhile 10 healthy women will be treated unnecessarily, and more than 200 "will experience important psychological distress including anxiety and uncertainty for years because of false positive findings."

Another nonprofit medical group, theNNT.com, has spelled out a disturbing implication of these data. (NNT stands for "number needed to treat," which refers to the number of people who must receive a treatment for one person to receive any benefit. Ideally, the number is 1.) The NNT notes that some overdiagnosed women might "die due to aggressive therapies such as chemotherapy and major surgery." Thus any benefit from screening "is balanced out by mortal harms from overdiagnosis and false-positives." Breast-cancer specialist Michael Baum, who helped found the United Kingdom's breast-screening program, has advocated abandoning such programs, which he believes might cut short more lives than they extend.

As for PSA tests, a federal task force of medical experts estimates that 1.3 deaths may be averted for every 1,000 men between the ages of 55 and 69 tested for 13 years. But for every man whose life is extended, many more will experience "false-positive results that require additional testing and possible prostate biopsy;

overdiagnosis and overtreatment; and treatment complications, such as incontinence and erectile dysfunction." A 2017 analysis by the task force estimated the ratio of beneficial PSA tests to false positives and overdiagnosis to be as high as 1/240.

A 2013 meta-analysis by Cochrane Group found "no significant reduction" in mortality resulting from PSA tests. "The strategy of routinely screening all men with PSA tests leads to interventions that are not saving lives and may be causing harm," the NNT stated. The discoverer of the prostate-specific antigen, pathologist Richard Ablin, has called the PSA test a "profit-driven public health disaster."

All-Cause Versus Specific Mortality and "Torturing the Data"

Studies of tests for a specific cancer generally look at mortality attributed to that cancer. Mammograms are thus deemed effective if women who get mammograms die less often *from breast cancer* than women who do not get mammograms. This method can overstate the benefits of tests, because it might omit deaths resulting, directly or indirectly, from the diagnosis. After all, surgery, chemotherapy and radiation can have devastating iatrogenic effects, including heart disease, opportunistic infections, other forms of cancer and suicide.

Therefore some studies measure "all-cause" mortality. A 2015 meta-analysis by epidemiologist John Ioannidis (renowned for bringing the scientific replication crisis to light) and others found no reductions in all-cause mortality from tests for cancer of the breast, prostate, colon, lung, cervix, mouth or ovaries for asymptomatic patients.

In a recent editorial in the *European Journal of Clinical Investigation*, Ioannidis and four co-authors argue that cancer screening (especially mammograms and PSA tests) does more harm than good and should be abandoned. They expect this proposal to be met with "fierce opposition." Screening they note, "is big business: more screening means more patients, more clinical revenue to diagnostic and clinical departments, and more survivors in need of care and follow-up."

Cancer boosters commonly point to improvements in survival rates, the length of time between diagnosis and death. Survival rates for some cancers have indeed grown as a result of more widespread and higher-resolution testing, which detects cancer earlier. But as a 2015 analysis points out, in general people do not live longer as a result of early detection. They simply live longer with a diagnosis of cancer, with all its harmful emotional, economic and physiological consequences.

Using survival rates to promote tests is an example of what critics of mammography have called "tortur[ing] the data to make it confess to what one knows to be the real truth." What the data on screening actually suggest is that millions of men and women have endured the trauma of cancer diagnoses and treatments unnecessarily. That strikes me as a case of monstrous malpractice.

Corruption in the Cancer Industry

The aggressive, can-do American approach to health care isn't working when it comes to medicine in general and cancer medicine in particular. The U.S. spends far more per capita on health care, including cancer care, than any other country, but higher expenditures have not led to longer lives. Quite the contrary. Europe, which spends much less on cancer care than the U.S., has lower cancer mortality rates, according to a 2015 study. So do countries such as Mexico, Italy and Brazil, according to Our World in Data.

The American approach fosters corruption. According to a 2019 essay in *Stat News* by oncologist Vinay Prasad, many cancer specialists accept payments from firms whose drugs they prescribe. This practice "leads us to celebrate marginal drugs as if they were game-changers," Prasad argues. "It leads experts to ignore or downplay flaws and deficits in cancer clinical trials. It keeps doctors silent about the crushing price of cancer medicines."

Last year *The New York Times* and *ProPublica* reported that top officials at Sloan Kettering Cancer Center "repeatedly violated policies on financial conflicts of interest, fostering a culture in which profits appeared to take precedence over research and patient care." Sloan Kettering's chief medical officer, Jose Baselga, "failed to disclose millions of dollars in payments from drug and health care companies in dozens of articles in medical journals." Baselga left Sloan Kettering to become head of cancer research at the drug firm AstraZeneca.

The desire of oncologists to produce monetizable findings might also compromise the quality of their research. A 2012 examination of 53 "landmark" cancer studies found that only six could be reproduced. The so-called Reproducibility Project: Cancer Biology has examined 14 more recent highly cited studies, and has confirmed only five without qualification.

Solution: Gentle Cancer Medicine?

So what's the solution to all these problems? Some health-care experts espouse "conservative medicine" as a way to reduce health-care costs and improve outcomes. In "The Case for Being a Medical Conservative," a manifesto published last year, four physicians (including the aforementioned Vinay Prasad) urge colleagues to recognize the human body's "inherent healing properties" and to acknowledge "how little effect the clinician has on outcomes." Physicians will thus protect themselves "against our greatest foe—hubris."

Medical conservatives happily adopt new therapies "when the benefit is clear and the evidence strong and unbiased," the authors emphasize, but many alleged advances "offer, at best, marginal benefits." Conservative cancer medicine, as I envision it, would engage in less testing, treatment, fear-mongering, military-style rhetoric and hype. It would recognize the limits of medicine, and it would honor the Hippocratic oath: First, do no harm.

Physicians cannot bring about a shift toward conservative cancer medicine on their own. We consumers must help them. We must recognize the limits of medicine and the healing capacities of our bodies. We must resist tests and treatments that have marginal benefits, at best. We may never cure cancer, which stems from the collision of our complex biology with entropy, the tendency of all systems toward disorder. But if we can curtail our fear and greed, our cancer care will surely improve.

A final note: I'd like to thank experts I've cited above–John Ioannidis, Siddhartha Mukherjee, Vinay Prasad, Azra Raza and Gilbert Welch–as well as Cochrane and theNNT.com for their blunt, courageous assessments of cancer medicine. People and groups like these represent our best hope for health-care reform. We just have to listen to them.

The views expressed are those of the author(s) and are not necessarily those of Scientific American.

Abou the Author

John Horgan, who has written for Scientific American *since 1986, comments on science on his free online journal Cross-Check. He has also posted his books* Mind-Body Problems *and* My Quantum Experiment *online. Horgan teaches at Stevens Institute of Technology.*

GLOSSARY

abberant Different from an agreed-upon standard.

benign Harmless or safe.

cell line A cell culture used in research, cultivated from the division and reproduction of a single cell.

cessation The act of terminating or ending something.

community hospital A general hospital primarily serving the health of a particular area, rather than also participating in research or training.

earmark To allocate or set aside for a specific purpose.

epidemiology A research discipline focusing on the appearance, causes, and patterns of a disease in a population.

immunotherapy A recently-developed form of cancer treatment that uses the body's own immune system to fight cancer.

malignant Dangerous or infectious.

metastasis The development of a cancer into growths beyond the original cancer site.

mastectomy The surgical removal of a breast.

mRNA vaccine A vaccine that uses ribonucleic acid (RNA) to train the body's immune response, rather than using a pathogen sample.

nucleotide A normal component of DNA that may play a role in cancer development.

oncology A medical discipline devoted specifically to treating cancer.

petrochemical A chemical substance derived from petroleum.

precipitous Sudden and significant.

preliminary An initial instance in advance of a more definitive version.

randomized controlled trial A standard procedure for evaluating new treatments, based on randomly-chosen participants to join a control group or receive the treatment.

screening A test or survey for a possible illness.

suboptimal Less than ideal in performance on a particular metric.

tumor An excess growth of a particular tissue, which may be malignant or benign.

FURTHER INFORMATION

"Cancer." Our World in Data, https://ourworldindata.org/cancer.

"The History of Cancer." American Cancer Society, https://www.cancer.org/cancer/understanding-cancer/history-of-cancer.html.

"What Is Cancer?" National Cancer Institute, https://www.cancer.gov/about-cancer/understanding/what-is-cancer.

Geggel, Laura. "If Dogs Can Smell Cancer, Why Don't They Screen People?" *Scientific American*, December 27, 2017, https://www.scientificamerican.com/article/if-dogs-can-smell-cancer-why-dont-they-screen-people/.

Habr, Dany. "We Must End Ageism in Cancer Clinical Trials." *Scientific American,* June 14, 2022, https://www.scientificamerican.com/article/we-must-end-ageism-in-cancer-clinical-trials/.

Kessler, Rebecca. 'Air Pollution's Impact on Cancer Is "Grossly Underestimated'." *Scientific American*, July 1, 2014, https://www.scientificamerican.com/article/air-pollution-s-impact-on-cancer-is-grossly-underestimated/.

Small, Leah. "What the FDA Ruling about 'Dense Breasts' Means for Cancer Risk and Screening." *Scientific American*, April 10, 2023, https://www.scientificamerican.com/article/what-the-fda-ruling-about-dense-breasts-means-for-cancer-risk-and-screening/.

Wallis, Claudia. "Deadly Spread of Some Cancers May Be Driven by a Common Mouth Microbe." *Scientific American*, October 1, 2020, https://www.scientificamerican.com/article/deadly-spread-of-some-cancers-may-be-driven-by-a-common-mouth-microbe/.

CITATIONS

1.1 Cancerous Coconspirators: Tumor Cells That Travel Together Spread Cancer by Viviane Callier (April 1, 2016); 1.2 Close-Up Views of Tumors Reveal a New Cancer Biology by Philip Ball (April 21, 2020); 1.3 How Evolution Helps Us Understand Cancer and Control It by Athena Aktipis (January 1, 2021); 1.4 The Colon Cancer Conundrum by Cassandra Willyard (December 1, 2021); 1.5 How to Tell whether a Cancer Is Caused by Plain Bad Luck by Viviane Callier (April 26, 2022); 2.1 Experimental Blood Test Detects Cancer up to Four Years before Symptoms Appear by Rachel Nuwer (July 21, 2020); 2.2 Taking Early Cancer Detection to the Next Level by Joshua J. Ofman, Azra Raza (November 1, 2020); 2.3 The COVID Cancer Effect by Usha Lee McFarling (December 1, 2021); 2.4 Most People at Risk for Lung Cancer Never Get Screened: Here's How to Fix That by Simar Bajaj (September 6, 2022); 2.5 When Should You Get a Mammogram? by Lauren J. Young (June 2, 2023); 3.1 Do Cellphones Cause Cancer? Probably, but It's Complicated by Christopher J. Portier, Wendy L. Leonard (June 13, 2016); 3.2 One More Pioneering Woman in Science You've Probably Never Heard of by Ellen Elliott (November 6, 2017); 3.3 Pancreatic Cancer Vaccine Shows Promise in Small Initial Trial by Tanya Lewis (May 11, 2023); 3.4 Having Their Fallopian Tubes Removed Will Spare a Large Number of Women from Ovarian Cancer by Joseph V. Sakran, Kara Long Roche, Rebecca Stone (May 21, 2023); 3.5 Adjusting Your Body Clock May Stave Off Cancer by Lydia Denworth (July 1, 2023); 4.1 Scientists Tackle Lethal Childhood Brain Cancer by Esther Landhuis (October 28, 2016); 4.2 A Shot against Cancer by Karen Weintraub (December 1, 2016); 4.3 Are We Innately Immune to Cancer? by Mark Lowdell (January 24, 2019); 4.4 Darwin's Ideas on Evolution Drive a Radical New Approach to Cancer Drug Use by James DeGregori, Robert Gatenby (August 1, 2019); 5.1 We Must Improve Equity in Cancer Screening by Melba Newsome (December 1, 2021); 5.2 The Race to Stop a Plastics Plant Scores a Crucial Win by Judith Enck, Rebekah Creshkoff (September 23, 2022); 5.3 Clinical Trials Have the Best Medicine but Do Not Enroll the Patients Who Need It by David H. Freedman (January 1, 2019); 5.4 The Cancer Industry: Hype vs. Reality by John Horgan (February 12, 2020).

Each author biography was accurate at the time the article was originally published.

INDEX

S

T

V

W

Y